Silence = Death

The Infectious Lie of HIV/AIDS

By

Niles Stanley

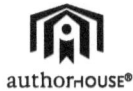

authorHOUSE®

AuthorHouse™
1663 Liberty Drive, Suite 200
Bloomington, IN 47403
www.authorhouse.com
Phone: 1-800-839-8640

First published by AuthorHouse 7/25/2007

ISBN: 978-1-4343-1903-6 (sc)

Printed in the United States of America
Bloomington, Indiana

This book is printed on acid-free paper.

I am dedicating this book to Ed my friend and lover who died of AIDS. Since HIV/AIDS is of artificial origin made in a laboratory and diseased by politics many more people have lost life on many more levels. Up until recently I was not able to fully understand guilt by fear of the manmade political designer diseases that have no reason or respect for life past, present or future. I want to apologize to Ed for love lost between us due in part by fear of love and I realize now Ed forgives me from above. I want to also dedicate this book to my friends Bob, Ken and Wayne as well as friends at Boom, Ramrod, Alibi, Cubby Hole, Jackhammer and Java Boys in Ft. Lauderdale, Fl. allowing me to silently vent without much hassle. Without friends I would not be here today.

Preface

The enclosed information is just a segment of the complete story regarding the Bush Administration and co-sponsors of disease distribution affecting humanity. It has been extremely difficult to even get the enclosed information to the publisher with communication interferences being common place infiltrated onto my computer daily along with varying degrees of daily harassments. In addition, editing has been virtually impossible and as a result please excuse any stumblings of sentence structure or placement of data. The intent of this book is to raise awareness regarding the HIV/AIDS charade and reversed HIV/AIDS awareness to include humanity and not laboratory viral gene products being designed to trample on society and distributed by the current Bush Administration and co-sponsors of Globalization grappling for world control. New awareness is desperately needed for humanity to survive being blind-sided reversing spiritual love of nature and life. Humanity is being forgotten with twists of church and state owning spirituality becoming more and more sterility with less zest for life unable to live outside the confines of Silence = Death everywhere there is church and state and HIV/AIDS.

We need to become aware of the business of health wrapped in politics and put under a microscope a true analysis of what savvy means to the health of a person trying to dodge the bullet of unscrupulous business practices in health care by lethal Vaccine and Medicine Initiatives called HIV/AIDS. Layers upon more viruses in syringes and medicine to stigmatize and bury entire communities while grief carries us on is not living. Silence = Death while living and individuality with better ideas regarding living should be untangled from our current surrounding environment of protruding silence with death and dying prevailing in our lives to begin to heal in clarity what has been happening over the past decades living within an environment of lethal political ignorance practicing distributing death and dying labeling people HIV/AIDS. The government and co-sponsor's agendas of confusion and destroying healthy living will never end unless Silence = Death is understood to end the unnecessary violence once and for all the truth to be understood for healthier healing with more productive lives to live.

A life judged to live justified is not living having to walk on pins and needles while continually being HIV tested and harassed escalating unnecessary twisted anxiety over the period of a lifetime. Battering rhetoric conclusions of evidenced based lies regarding populations judged and deemed "high risk" is insane and dangerously unhealthy for everyone to swim in societal consequences of polluted politics and money perpetuating the big business of HIV/AIDS. Unfortunately, the reality today is we are living smaller within cruel political requirements to live in advertised justification being surrounded by hateful strategies of population and behavior control. And especially under the Bush Administration of increased upside down AIDS agendas and targeting practices to more frequently include women and minorities increasing anxiety into our lives. Money controlling people by viruses labeled HIV "high risk" people scopes of tunnel vision today is the twisted political right to our lives to target and harass vast numbers of people designated to die of HIV/AIDS using money today to cover up the truth of the disease labeled HIV/AIDS causing wide scale discrimination complications.

Politics is so disgustingly alarming for government to underhandedly judge people by a despicable right to our lives being controlled by their viral monies allotted for judging rights of inequality denying many people a life. Nobody should have to worry about living justified especially when there is no wide spread awareness to justify dodging the dangerous health care bullet of the Bush Administration and co-sponsors of death and dying. The Bush Administration and co-sponsors of corporate citizenship and evil population control strategies today is sad having to justify our existence by standards of gregarious arrogant evil rights to life entities precariously owning people.

The new disease creations by newly forming genetic engineering combinations the Bush Administration and co-sponsors are emerging into society ranging anywhere from Avian Flu to Small Pox to Sars and calling the diseases HIV/AIDS along with twisted strategies of awareness concentrating efforts and collaborating wasting time and lives of humans and animals in time is generating a society of vaccine and medicine outlets around the world encoding societal debilitation dependant upon government and corporations to ruin our lives. Encoding viruses into the world to validate a population "high risk" is genocide control strategies emerging stigma and disease as the status quo is cause for grave alarm. Vaccines and medicines infecting innocent people with political undertows of a twisted right to a life to destroy is disgustingly sad today labeling people persistently infected as a result of an HIV test complete with behavior regimens of medicine intake and bedroom check lists of safety is not valuing life or death controlled by paper monopoly money of no value whatsoever in the big business of HIV/AIDS the lie.

The Bush Administrations strategies as a business acting pretending their societal treatment initiatives are healthy is in reality causing pain and heartache by the millions under ominous political control. The right winged master plan to gain individual, community, population and world control is not proper protocol for real health around the world to communicate out in the open without worrying about being targeted. We need to eliminate the delusional power of the Bush Administration's escalating agendas of world control by disease, war and stigma. In fact, we are as a society just one or two more vaccination bundles away from unscrupulous health care business practices being forever out of control creating global corporate citizens with and without jobs to be further controlled by stigma and labels of individuality of family businesses being put into graves. If globalization continues its rampage of eliminating innocent individuals people and controlling citizens will soon be required to line up and be science projects for more people to walk around with disease advertising more fear causing more globalized discrimination and loneliness of a different business never ending Silence = Death. If we could be allowed to simply communicate instead of being gobbled up by the Bush monster machine rusty in oil of strategies increasing propagating Silence = Death and disease then we could end Silence = Death and disease and war.

The government and research experimentation schemes with business initiatives being enacted against individuals to be pseudo corporate citizens behaved by firm hand viruses in America and abroad with no choices whatsoever in life being human robots are schemes of infections and labels controlling society by upside down HIV/AIDS awareness. Cultures being put into test tubes isolating individuals to be trapped drowning in someone else's judgement is instilling lost time forced to learn an unhealthy foreign language of behavior control and labels as signs of the times as just the way it is in business success of executive power judging and eliminating life to be sad living in a right winged political environment of such hostility towards humanity.

HIV labels caused by various genetically engineered viral strains of viruses inclusive of bacteria and chemicals being packaged with genetically altered cross species cells all combined to create varying degrees of virulence used to sicken and label people as HIV/AIDS is causing humanity to rot. Individual genes being genetically altered by genetically engineered viruses causing more discrimination and hate crimes to emerge and be handed down into second and third generations and beyond deformations of society without a healthy course is sad to explain Silence = Death. Disease labeled HIV/AIDS is excruciatingly painful being silently altered and controlled right before our eyes. A government and corporate world nightmare together and separating from the world as individuals losing individuality losing energy to live as humans is a shame people are not made aware of the autrocities occuring at an escalated pace under the Bush Administration. Concluding disease as a consequence of behavior advertised as a deviant unhealthy act yet not of the person but of government and co-sponsors acting on behalf of the big business of HIV/AIDS is pure evil greed and selfish corruptness owning people dwindling while creating more land space to occupy.

Behaviors being surgically removed and dissected from individuals labeled "high risk" by genetically engineered viruses is a nightmare not to associate with a person and cruel and unusual creating fear to freeze the masses for everyone to be potential targets of disease propagation and isolation on many levels. The Bush Administration and co-sponsors of disease distribution as a fear strategy while standing on ceremony to establish corporate citizenship and globalization as a way of life is terrible place for America and around the world to always be judged by a few political monsters as a way of life and not a future especially in Silence = Death being the status quo. Annoying political behavior traits as strategies against the Bill of Rights unable to Act-Up under the current political environment of protesting with consequences by a corrupt Bush Administration has not been America for a long time. Government and corporate sponsorship of disease progression is a deafening loud cover up. Not one ounce of a voice contained by don't ask don't tell jargon equals more silence equals more death and no power to the people threatened by fear and stigma mantras forever controlling populations to behave as a result of viral money being infused into their business schemes of death and dying eliminating more people to control more people and more Silence = Death and more land space to waste and steel more nature and time with nature. Virus violence directing life to be dead under the rug is a constant "house cleaning" item for the Bush Administration and co-sponsors of disease propagation and don't ask don't tell slavery mantras to evil as sterile globalization is the reality today of manmade war and disease being covered up. A complete demise of individuality being covered by outward behaviors is a globalized business plan of disease distribution to control communities and countries installing fear of friends and family eliminated labeled "high risk" being a business item by cold blood extractions from mother earth growing colder in oil is burning real life today. Terrorism is being contained in silence of Silence = Death infiltrating into lives today not save by a right to life today living and labeled with HIV/AIDS the charade and terrorized by the system of disease awareness is pure terror especially when the disruptive system of Globalization is not being discussed yet war is discussed today and everyday as the status quo.

Human totals by evil unaccountable for nothing with no compassion behind their government/corporate sheltered hog houses filled with their unintelligible grunts of pig to bird species viruses being genetically engineered combining into Avian type flu bugs labeled HIV/AIDS where anything can happen scenarios blaming a person behaving badly in their test tube coop in terror. The proverbial enigma of Silence = Death nobody wants to discuss because of tears and fears today of the Bush Administration's strategic consequences infrastructure is to blame for their blatant attacks to extract, target and infect selected individuals, communities and countries to go unnoticed and ignored by criminal biological warfare under the table agendas of genocide and globalization. The Bush Administration and co-sponsors of laboratory disease propagation exploratory in the planning stages today of increasing an infrastructure to swiftly vaccinate vast numbers of individuals with live and attenuated viruses is the reality today of government and industry escalating genetic engineering combinations of species and chemicals to cross infect people. HIV/SIV/SHIV with any a myriad of other additives of Avian Flu, West Nile Virus, Sars, Ebola, Venezuelan Equine Virus, or even Anthrax to name a few is currently taking place within a global vaccine initiative.

Why not start with ending HIV/AIDS the enigma to end the stigma of disease emergence creating violence and heartache? The Bush Administration using viral war today for pure real life torture in loss of innocence altering the planet to be bitter stratified cement suffocated one level at a time at least needs a vote against war. If the devastation is allowed to continue life will not only equate to starting the day with an alarm for all life in nature will begin and end with many alarms by way of many more leveling wars and more Silence = Death on the horizon sweltering globalization sweat shops rising off the cement every second of the day. We as humans are part of the animal world trying to do the best we can, yet in the unnatural world of the Bush Administration and co-sponsors of globalization we are fortunate if we can do anything under their forced control to demise humanity trying the "best they can" creating difficulties and compromises of immunity by agendas in the beginning stages of vaccinating vast numbers of individuals. Military compromising natural immunity of spirit and body physically is tragic being labeled vulnerable "hardest hit" Gay community minorities consistently consequently compromised and disenfranchised. Life is difficult enough the way it is in America without the Bush Administration meddling destruction into our lives causing interruptions to confuse our natural immunity trying the best a person can be feeling freedom inside. The so-called American Patriot Acts uncivilized are forcing servants of their government and corporate destruction by fear and terror is sad with no real choices for freedom today from paper money controlling our every motional move inside and out. It is sad the Bush Administration abuses people by abusing money to cause pain causing more people to be infected by a system of Silence = Death with no healing by releasing the cure for disease labeled HIV/AIDS being unnecessary terror inside and out.

What really is the best anyone can be especially if ill with laboratory disease called HIV/AIDS a trap forcing don't ask don't tell Silence = Death wounded physically and spiritually by viral wars encapsulating the person as deserving of death and dying as the norm? Many are frustrated spiritually with the decimating crap of Federated America escalating a class system of discrimination tearing US apart in more ways than one. How can anyone be the best under the reality of Silence = Death and don't ask don't tell the unfairness of the debilitating system of disease distribution and stigma? Labels of people being forced upon all people incorrect ideals of HIV/AIDS is on the upside down AIDS awareness poster reading dead or alive. American style labeling complexities of cruelty is boring of incorrectly being disenfranchised as an American not a member of the corporate citizen uncivilized world. The heartache of internal silence is unhealthy not to say a word about the HIV/AIDS charade yet hate begets hate with violence apathy and political compliance complacency especially when the growing hate is forced by money twisting nature being forced evolution by genetically engineered viruses and chemicals.

Gender violence being subjective in America within the mantra prayer of "never hit a female" is a notion to imagine violence outside of a gender. Why hit anyone or imagine violence or tell someone they cannot defend themselves being glued to don't ask don't tell mantras within the repugnance of America that is barbaric and uncivilized? What is freedom of speech or expression in America anyway? Why allow individuals labeled civilian or otherwise compromised to be put into a military box of hate and violence because of military American lame excuses of morality being who is anyone who cannot ask or tell of the punishment living with Silence = Death? Military America is just so innately immorally cruel. Why hit anyone within the "hardest hit" communities of stigma, disease and hate crimes when learning and education would be a better path towards unity all inclusive of sexuality as an energy source to welcome more love and less war? The auspices of internal silences and sadness already being ripped torn today needs healing to defend Out Loud in the open for the best anyone can be not to be hit at all.

Federation America needs more social scorn of external and internal battering and less on mantras of don't ask don't tell, high risk "hardest hit" communities or hit anyone except a woman. Why not transparency to end of the external and internal violence felt being punished in the closet of HIV/AIDS surrounding the person feeling the bruises to reverse discrimination to be more sensitive for the truth to end Silence = Death. The closet in the military bleeding into so-called civilian life viewed as a target to nourish the closet of unannounced Military America today currently being mainstreamed around individuals for the "person" to be an issue of disease and behavior "issues" for society being forced into military freestyle violence matches of domestic and international hate crimes of no consequence in convictions not being labeled hate crimes because of political leveraging. Military style America with criminal political tactics of more and more violence against

Americans is becoming the status quo under the Bush years. Silence = Death to be a better human frustrated losing friends and family is a nightmare dream so frighteningly close yet so far away to dream for inclusiveness in prayers to become reality for healing in society not to be afraid to ask or tell. Today pure inequality to be the best anyone can be is Bushwacked and forced into the closet of don't ask don't tell Silence = Death. The forced closet is unable to stop the prayers for equality to remove internalizing military debauchery overwhelming the senses making no sense at all why we cannot convict the Bush Administration of hate crimes unpublicized decimating and destructive under the table political actions.

Being Gay is not a crime yet inequality disables our ability to grow and destroy the installed societal hate in the American atmosphere today to have the opportunity to transform tolerance into acceptance on the natural ground. "Be All That You Can Be" only in military terms of "Be All The Military Wants You To Be" or what the Bush Administration demands quiet and no questions asked of substance or meaning so boring and not real living in Federated America. Health gives more meaning to life than the current "America" under the Bush Administration giving real harassments for real grief in real time in their atmosphere of disease and fear of people mislabeled HIV/AIDS creating deeper frustrations, discontentment and greater heartache alone and disassembled. America today is a terrible place to live and die being harassed into isolation from cradle to grave just for being a minority targeted with a laboratory disease to "be all anyone can be" living in America today the land of bloody closets and secrets of distributed pain.

A Report titled Plenery Discussion - Future Directions located at www.nih.gov says;
Appropriate animal models determine the risks associated with specific organ transplants from specific animals and cooperation between corporate entities and multiple laboratories will accelerate the development in this field and create the kind of open research environment that is more likely than an environment with competitive secrecy to convince the public that science is sound.

(Specific animals such as monkeys that have been exploited to continue the secret facade of HIV/AIDS by the cooperation of formalized secret pacts between government, corporate entities and multiple laboratories around the world forcing the acceleration of the HIV/AIDS field to include more players hiding more secrets about the big

business of HIV/AIDS will not end until we reverse HIV/AIDS Awareness ending Silence = Death.)

The Report titled; The Genomic Revolution: Unveiling The Unity of Life

http://books.nap.edu/books/0309074363/html/34.html
Says;

Benefits are a counterweight to the concerns voiced about the misuse of genetic

information. The fact that science is a human instrument one that can be used wisely or foolishly and only an informed public will decide what will happen.

A Report titled HIV Vaccines & Human Rights
www.avac.org/pdf/primer/humanrights.pdf

For large scale human trials to be successful in skeptical populations, it will be important for trial volunteers to have confidence that the candidate vaccine going into their arms is the most promising product science can currently produce for efficacy testing rather than an experimental agent chosen for testing because lack of public or private investment left few options.

A Report
AIDS Vaccine Fails to Show Efficacy in Thai Trial located
www.avac.org/AIDSVAXthai.htm
Says;

Now is the time to reinvigorate AIDS vaccine research yet there are no real plans to make an AIDS vaccine universally accessible.

A Report
NIH AIDS Research Program Evaluation Vaccine Research & Development Area Review Panel Findings and Recommendations
  http://www.nih.gov/od/oar/public/pubs/vaccine.pdf
Says;

One significant concern is the present lack of basic knowledge needed by private enterprise to meaningfully enter the AIDS vaccine development. Another concern is despite proof of principle in some nonhuman primate models a widespread perception that an effective vaccine against HIV is highly unlikely and will be extremely difficult to develop and is far in the future.

The Report titled "AIDS Vaccine Fails to Show Efficacy in Thai Trial" located at www.avac.org/AIDSVAXthai.htm Says;

Sometimes the results from clinical trials will be disappointing, but all of us need to be prepared for the long haul to find a vaccine against the biggest infectious disease killer.

The Report
A Partnership for Health: Minorities and Biomedical Research www.niaid.nih.gov/publications/minorityhealth.pdf under the heading Microbiology and Infectious Diseases

Says;
The microbiology and Infectious diseases segment of NIAID's agenda includes research to control and prevent diseases in humans caused by virtually every infectious agent except HIV. NIAID supports a wide spectrum of projects ranging from basic biomedical research to clinical trials to evaluate potential drugs and vaccines and NIAID currently supports clinical studies seeking to expand recruitment of minority populations into these studies.

The Jordan Report www.niaid.nih.gov/dmid/vaccines/jordan20/jordan20_2002.pdf

HIV vaccine research always has been an integral part of NIAID's research portfolio with the goal of identifying a vaccine.In the last 7 years the program has received an influx of funds enabling it to grow exponentially.

A Report
Genomic Revolution: Unveiling The Unity of Life http://books.nap.edu/books/0309074363/html/196.html
Says;

Genetic information can be used to classify and lump, split and separate, identify and admit. Many nations have granted the right of return if you can show that your ancestors come from a particular place. Citizenship oftentimes keys on biological inheritance. In the future genetics will interest those social, scientific, anthropological, and even archeological areas in very interesting ways.

The National Institutes of Health Fiscal Year 2003 Plan For HIV-Related Research www.oar.nih.gov/public/pubs/fy2003/iii_etiology.pdf

ETIOLOGY AND PATHOGENESIS
NIH Fiscal Year 2003 Plan for HIV-Related Research
Says;

Since the initial isolation of HIV in 1983 and its identification as the causative agent of AIDS tremendous progress has been made in understanding the genetic structure and variability of the viral genome and the critical aspects of the virus life cycle as well as the functions of viral gene products and their interaction with the host.

The Report
Making the Case for Genetics: Roles for the Public Health Laboratory" Meeting Summary October 20, 2003, Washington DC Hosted by the Association of Public Health Laboratories and the Centers for Disease Control and Prevention www.phppo.cdc.gov/dis/pdf/genetics/summaryreport.pdf

Says;

Knowledge of the biology of infectious agents and not the host has thus far been the most important factor to infection, disease progression, vaccine efficacy, and treatment success.

In time the system will be able to use knowledge of host factors to identify persons and populations more likely to become infected, manifest serious disease and benefit or be harmed by treatments and vaccines.

The National Institutes of Health Fiscal Year 2003 Plan For HIV-Related Research www.oar.nih.gov/public/pubs/fy2003/iii_etiology.pdf
ETIOLOGY AND PATHOGENESIS
NIH Fiscal Year 2003 Plan for HIV-Related Research

Says;

Host factors or the particular nature of the host response plays a critical role in determining whether and when disease arises following infection.

Research at the cellular and molecular levels includes studies of mechanisms by which HIV infects various cell types as well as the interaction between the viral regulatory elements and host cell factors that appear to be directed at maintaining a persistent infection and the viral and host mediated mechanisms that influence the level of viral expression seen in successive stages of HIV disease. Continued support of in vivo research (in human research) is a high priority at NIH in order to further an understanding of the interaction between the virus and host immune system responses.
NIH-sponsored cohort studies constitute a major resource for pathogenesis research.
Specific cohorts such as long term nonprogressors, HIV-exposed but uninfected individuals, and rapid progressors will provide clues for treatment and vaccine research by helping to characterize immune

response profiles and by providing information on correlates of immunity.

Some of the studies that examine gender differences compare factors other than sex in patients. HIV-infected women are more likely to be poor, to belong to racial minorities, to be of poor health status, and use injection drugs. These are all factors that might have important effects on health outcomes for both men and women infected with HIV.

(The knowledge of the biology of infectious agents and not the host has thus far been the most important contributory factor to infection disease progression and vaccine efficacy. However, host factors or the particular nature of the host response plays a critical role in determining whether and when disease arises following vaccine induced infections because the viruses are being encoded into genetic structure to abuse classifying, lumping, splitting, separating and identifying certain individuals or special populations. Abusive treatment success has been the design of the evil Vaccine Enterprise and the HIV/AIDS charade from the start manipulating the viruses as well as animals and humans as incubators to propagate disease and stigmatization strategies. The Bush Administration and co-sponsors of death and dying only care about the in vivo human and animal "hosts" as carriers of government and industry bacteria and viruses to end life for their purposes of control. The abuse of "hosts" as slaves to internally mutate their lab viruses and bacteria to increase disease and discrimination against various populations pitting one against another is the most diabolical part of the mutating genetic engineering processes. Human and animal hosts to propagate more human and animal devastation yet to be unleashed on the world by an ignorant agenda harboring biological hazardous materials is scary politically motivated Bushwacked business today. The selected hosts have been previously targeted to receive lab generated "infectious agents" that are designed to encode diseases of a particular cause and affect to ravage and stigmatize a community with decimating wasting syndromes or Kaposis Sarcoma as outcomes of strategic targeting disenfranchised selected "hosts" rather it be injection drug users, Gay men or poor women as a start to more and more strategies and more selected "populations" being forced into a quagmire of demeaning layers and labels to where disease, stigma and wasting is becoming status quo designed to engulf vast numbers of individuals with grief and pain. The agenda of the Bush Administration and co-sponsors of discrimination and isolation trying to establish an environmental infrastructure to disable more people to be labeled so-called "minority" using HIV drugs, or poor for more social control over people is insanely sad. Targeting and recruiting individuals into "high risk" lethal HIV clinical trials designed to create more fear and societal control is layering insanely sad on an escalated level and needs to be stopped immediately. The hate mongers including financial status as a host contributory factor important to disease progression is increasingly sad segregating people into financial compartments to target first hand media hype bought and paid by industry sponsors layering disseminating lies and stories of super natant mutations to alarm people as different is excruciating pain. The Bush Administration and co-sponsors of homelessness ideals torturing the same people already inflicted with their gross societal pain being labeled "high risk" societal lepers needs to be stopped immediately. Painful layers upon labels and more labels upon more layers in the big business of HIV/AIDS the charade is disgustingly alarming.)

A Report
NIH AIDS Research Program Evaluation Vaccine Research & Development Area Review Panel Findings and Recommendations
http://www.nih.gov/od/oar/public/pubs/vaccine.pdf

Says;

Safety concerns continue to cloud the development of attenuated virus vaccines for human use but not efficacy. Guidelines should be established for advancement of a vaccine product to efficacy trials sponsored by the NIH, although the precise criteria might vary with the concept under evaluation.

A Report
Therapeutic HIV Vaccines: Things to Consider http://www.the-body.com/pinf/vaccines.html

Says;

The type of virus used to infect the animals in the studies might also make a difference in terms of applicability to the human setting and that animals used in other studies do not develop disease following infection with HIV so researchers have been less enthused about the results of studies where infection was blocked in animals to the human setting.

(Safety is clouding the intrepid HIV clinical trials of efficacy of upside down treatment success where success means a hidden infection where infection blocked by animals in the eyes and hearts of scientists and researchers is a sad day. The Bush Administration and co-sponsors of the HIV/AIDS charade supporting certain researchers and scientists are not enthused when infections are blocked by natural immunity so they are designing more effective invasive strategies to ensure vaccine induced viral infections.)

A Report
National Institute for Health Fiscal Year 2001 Plan for HIV-Related Research located at www.nih.gov/od/oar/public/pubs/fy2001pln
Says;

Mechanisms of action of vaccine adjuvants and enhanced modes of HIV and related lentivirus antigen presentation is to induce different cytokine responses and carry out translational research in non-human primates and human vaccinees.

The Report
Panel Session I: Cross-Species Transmission – Species Specificity and Tropism http://www.niaid.nih.gov/dait/cross-species/page3.htm
Says;

It has been observed that many large complex viruses have evolved genetic mechanisms for modulating immune responses that would otherwise attack them. Some of them carry genes that block tumor necrosis factor induction of infected cell apoptosis.

The Report titled

The current Status of HIV-1 Vaccine Development, 2004: Recomendations for the Future by The NIAID AIDS Vaccine Research Working Group www.niaid.nih.gov/daids/vaccine/pdf/AVRWG/final-report.pdf

Says;

There is no consensus among investigators as to what ENV sequence to select as the basis of immunogenicity design. Decisions taken are generally based on rational, defensible principles, but easily could turn out to be mistakes. In addition, the article says emerging research information suggests choosing wild-type HIV-1 genes from a country where a vaccine is to be tested is not necessary. Knowledge needs to be gained in this area to better guide the decisions that have long-term and expensive consequences.

The report

Vaccine Concepts/Designs http://www.niaid.nih.gov/daids/vaccine/pseudovirions.htm

Says;

Identify additional HIV isolate(s) that retain sufficient envelope glycoprotein to mimic wild-type HIV to generate a pseudovirion vaccine.

The Report located at http://www.thebody.com/niaid/2004/hiv vaccine.html

Titled -

Methods to Enhance Immune Responses to HIV

Developing Immune Responses

Says;

B lymphocytes (B cells) produce antibodies to a specific foreign invader like HIV or a vaccine.

A Report

National Institute for Health Fiscal Year 2001 Plan for HIV-Related Research located at www.nih.gov/od/oar/public/pubs/fy2001pln.pdf

Says;

Multivalent vaccine candidates incorporating different genetic clades and antigentic types to increase breadth of immune responses.

A Report titled The Centers For Disease Control HIV/STD/TB Prevention News Update Dated July 11, 2002 located a www.thebody.com/cdc/news_updates_archive/july11_02/aids_vaccine.html

or www.thebody.com

Says;

A protective vaccine potentially containing hundreds or thousands of viral samples would be impossible to test and manufacture and may not be tolerated by humans.

Dr. Margaret Johnson, head of the National Institutes of Health's AIDS Vaccine Program, noted that nobody really knows how common superinfection may be and vaccine researchers assumed that an effective vaccine would have to be made up of samples of each of the major seven or eight classes of HIV now circulating around the world.

A Report

Progress in HIV Vaccine Research located at www.blackwell-synergy.com

Says;

Studies of HIV vaccines in animal models are essential for the selection of a vaccine, or combination of vaccines and will only be possible through clinical trials in human volunteers. However, the issues surrounding clinical efficacy trials of HIV vaccines are many including ethical issues, true informed consent, lack of coercion, protection of confidentiality and the fact that the patient will test positive for antibodies to HIV.

A Bulletin
Bulletin of ExperimentalTreatments for AIDS
Summer/Autumn 2001
A Publication of the San Francisco AIDS Foundation
AIDS Vaccines: The Ethical and Social Issues http://www.thebody.com/sfaf/summer01/vaccines.html#harm
Says;

Positive antibody tests are a predictable and extremely serious consequence of participation in a vaccine trial, it is accepted that researchers must not only warn participants of the issue but actively assist them in dealing with its ramifications. Researchers suggest to volunteers is to alert them up front so they can help them proactively rather than after a problem has happened. Depending on the circumstances, researchers may provide volunteers with a letter explaining their test results with whoever needs an explanation.

Immigration issues are a particular worry, since a positive HIV antibody test can threaten a person's ability to remain in the U.S. Clinicians have a little more ability at times with insurance companies and jobs, but the Immigration and Naturalization Service (INS) is sort of an entity unto itself, Dr. Buchbinder explains. They are the most unreasonable people and their constituency is a completely powerless group. Colleagues at NIH have alluded that they will do everything in their power, but there are certain things that they don't have control over.

In some cases the legal and social stigma may be so severe as to make certain research impossible for example, in countries where laws against homosexual behavior are so strict and actively enforced that MSM can never safely come forward. Even in less oppressive environments, researchers must take into account the vulnerability of populations they study and make every effort to minimize harm.

The question seemed particularly urgent a few years ago when official guidelines requested early treatment. The Declaration of Helsinki stated flatly that in any medical study every patient including those of a control group should be assured of the best proven diagnostic and therapeutic method. If HAART is the standard of medical care it must be available to any vaccinees who become infected, however poor, and wherever they live. One critical issue is the possibility that uninfected vaccinees will test positive on HIV antibody tests due to antibodies stimulated by the vaccine. This can cause problems in a variety of areas, from insurance policies to immigration issues. They warn about this possibility, Dr. Buchbinder says and the clinicians go through a very extensive education piece before we enroll anybody.... They ask them about the potential for their needing to be tested in a variety of different kinds of settings in the future and whether or not this could have a negative impact.

(The clinical trials that predictably generate HIV positive test results in a large number of clinical trial participants being altered physically and personally. The resulting grave and serious consequences leave individuals dependent on researchers that may provide volunteers with a letter explaining their test results or speak with whoever needs an explanation is a lie and a cover-up to the consequences of the life altering experience. The only "circumstance" is testing HIV positive due to the vaccinations in the clinical trial, and what the NIH is saying is each individual has a circumstance contingent on behavior, and if the behavior is deemed letter qualified then a letter will be generated on behalf of that particular individual even though the individual is still HIV positive and infected. The letter does not secure a job, insurance, travel or whoever needs an explanation from the government.

In addition, immigration issues are a particular worry, since a positive HIV antibody test can threaten a person's ability to remain in the U.S. with no letter available from the Immigration and Naturalization Service since the National Institute of Health as a middle person gives a lame excuse saying they will try to do everything in our power, but there are certain things that they just don't really have control over are again lies since the Bush Administration can allow anyone they want to remain in America regardless of what the government Immigration Department says. The government, unfortunately, has control over practically everything. Imagine coming to America from another country, and possibly spending a life savings to get here, and once settled in America someone as an immigrant is targeted by deceptive recruiting efforts of the clinical trial infrastructure. And once an immigrant accepts participating in a HIV clinical trial the newly immigrated individual is unaware they have accepted participating in a trap of expulsion and a nightmare for life. The immigrant becomes HIV positive during the trial and then is immediately expelled from America without a letter. But that is just the beginning of the extremely serious consequences of participation in the vaccine trial system since being an immigrant and HIV positive the immigrant is requested to leave America. The nightmare gets worse for the immigrant, since the immigrant is carrying an infection labeled as HIV and the corresponding country may request a no right to return policy denying entry into the corresponding country or worse stranded with an infection with no place to turn to rest.

The disclosure information prior to enrollment in the clinical trial is full of lies. They ask them about the potential for someone needing to be tested in a variety of different types of settings in the future or whether or not that would be an inconvenience. The reality of the devastation of seroconversion of the majority of vaccinees targeted in the clinical trials is way beyond an inconvenience.)

A Report
Social Challenges in HIV Vaccine Development
http://www.cdc.gov/hiv/vaccine/vusocial.htm
Says;

Vaccine acceptance will require community education about vaccines in general of HIV/AIDS and the meaning of HIV antibody seropositive. In many cases acceptance will also require the building of trust with communities that have experienced exploitation by biomedical research in the past.

Testing preventive HIV vaccines presents numerous social challenges. For example, persons who are targeted for recruitment into large-scale phase III trials are likely to be drawn from communities that have been historically marginalized and disenfranchised where HIV is most prevalent. Targeted communities often strongly distrust of the federal government and public health research especially around the issue of HIV/AIDS. Also immunization may result in participants developing vaccine induced HIV antibodies. Because HIV antibody testing is sometimes a requirement for accessing insurance, medical care, and employment, trial participants may be exposed to discrimination based on antibody tests.

(The majority of vaccine candidates will engender an antibody response in vaccinees, causing trial volunteers to test positive on standard HIV antibody tests, and as a result a positive HIV test result leads to discrimination in health insurance, medical care, employment and social stigma to name a few ramifications resulting in many individuals being marginalized and disenfranchised from society. The simple fact of participating in an HIV vaccine trial may cause someone to be labeled high-risk individual, a gay person, or a drug user is exactly what the Bush Administration is striving to achieve since discrimination, creating stigma, labeling, isolating individuals and creating infections and disease is their expertise along with denying health insurance, jobs, traveling and housing because of a HIV antibody positive test and vaccine induced infection exemplifies the impoverished mind set of the Bush Administration eliminating democratic votes. Clinicians recruiting individuals knowing the vaccine engenders an antibody response signaling an infection caused by bacteria and/or a virus infecting, labeling and stigmatizing an individual with HIV inscriptions is unfortunately the heartless direction America is educating in HIV/AIDS awareness of discrimination and stigma as planned by the hate mongers of the Bush Administration and co-sponsors of death and dying. The testing technology verbiage manipulation stating their is a difference between vaccine induced infection and actual infection is a lie. It is all vaccine induced infection, but used as a diversion within the Vaccine Enterprise's manipulation terminology for recruitment purposes. However, the testing technology can distinguish between an HIV vaccine induced Semliki Forest Virus infection or a vaccine induced Venezuelan Equine Encephalitis virus, as well as Smallpox, Alpha viruses, Adenoviruses, Chimeric viruses or any of the other genetically engineered concoctions of viruses in a Global Virus Panel of pathogens collected around the world and being used in a variety of ways with inscriptions of HIV/AIDS tags to continue segregating, separating, and isolating amongst "special populations" and communities forced to dwindle in a box of disenfranchised disease with little or no care.)

The report titled;
National Institute for Health Fiscal Year 2001 Plan for HIV-Related Research located at www.nih.gov/od/oar/public/pubs/fy2001pln.pdf

Says;

Determine methods of achieving informed consent for vaccine efficacy trials and consider the endpoints particularly disease progression and clinical outcomes and benefits of long-term follow-up.

(The HIV/AIDS charade can manipulate their viruses being genetically engineered buy combining animal and human viruses to more closely go undetected or create illnesses swiftly during the HIV clinical trials dependent upon the adverse agendas of coercion to go undetected by naive populations. Laboratory adaptated viruses that resemble disease progression in so-called "High Risk" people coerced into signing informed consent agreements to die unnoticed.)

The National Institutes of Health Fiscal Year 2003 Plan For HIV-Related Research www.oar.nih.gov/public/pubs/fy2003/iii_etiology.pdf
ETIOLOGY AND PATHOGENESIS
NIH Fiscal Year 2003 Plan for HIV-Related Research
Says;

Since the initial isolation of HIV in 1983 and its identification as the causative agent of AIDS tremendous progress has been made in understanding genetic structure and variability of the viral genome, the critical aspects of the virus life cycle, and the functions of viral gene products along with their interaction with the host.

The Report titled Reagent Resource Support for AIDS Vaccine Development located at www.niaid.nih.gov/contract/archive/rfp0301.pdf

Says;

Reclone, subclone or modify vector constructs provided by the Project Officer for production of HIV, SIV, or SHIV gene products including those cloned from HIV-1 field isolates and use the altered constructs to produce HIV, SIV, or SHIV gene products.

A Report
Reagent Resource Support for AIDS Vaccine Development
www.niaid.nih.gov/contract/archive/rfp0301.pdf
The Division of Acquired Immune Deficiency Syndrome (DAIDS) of the National Institute of Allergy and Infectious Diseases (NIAID), National Institutes of Health (NIH) Says;

The highest priority of DAIDS is the discovery, development, and evolution of HIV/AIDS vaccines and other prevention products. Facilitating research of DAIDS has long provided the research community with standardized quality-controlled reagents through the National Institute of Health AIDS Research and Reference Reagent Program. Large evaluation units and HIV Vaccine Trials Network require large quantities of such reagents not available through the AIDS Research and Reference Reagent Program. To advance the development of both vaccine and non-vaccine prevention products DAIDS is seeking ways to generate and acquire reagents and technologies made available for sponsored AIDS vaccine research and development projects. Many such reagents are not commercially available and require customized production and quality control. Reagents required for this research include but are not limited to viral gene products and associated peptides, adjuvants, cytokines, virus stocks, expression vectors, monoclonal and polyclonal antibodies, and sometimes unforeseen but appropriately and timely produced reagents. DAIDS supports under contract currently a facility to produce or otherwise acquire these types of reagents for AIDS vaccine research. In addition DAIDS the contractor has the capability to store, maintain, assure quality control and distribute large quantities of reagents. Facilitating research and development of potential AIDS vaccines in preclinical and clinical studies is essential to continue the service. By the end of the fourth year of the contract provide a transition plan and implement an orderly transition of data, reagents, all government Furnished Property (GFP) and materials and specimens to a successor Contractor or to the Government, subject to Project Officer approval and shall deliver if requested by the Project Officer and by the completion date of the contract the following items: original date, reagents, stored specimens, virus stocks, and any necessary information related thereto an inventory of Government Furnished Property.

As specified by or as designated by the Project Officer obtain by purchase or other arrangement and then characterize individual viral gene products of HIV, SIV, SHIV or related human and nonhuman primate lentiviruses in each contract year and obtain field and laboratory isolates of HIV-1 or other related retroviruses from various sources. Genes for cloning into expression vectors and prepare or acquire all necessary materials for cloning genes into suitable cloning vectors. Grow, evaluate, and characterize genetically modified cloning vectors. Clone genes identified by the Project Officer into appropriate expression vectors. The selection and source of the DNA and vector used for cloning will be specified by the Project Officer and shall be acquired or produced by the contractor. Maintain an electronic inventory of reagent stocks and a database of all reagents analysis results. Provide Inventory and Database Management System and maintain a computerized inventory and distribution database to track samples and activities under the contract. Use shipping conditions appropriate to preserving activity of any reagent to comply with domestic and international postal regulations and pertinent regulation by international, national, and local entities for the transportation of hazardous materials, including infectious substances. Commercial carriers airlines and couriers i.e. FedEx, DHL, and others can also impose conditions to their acceptance of packages for transports within the United States. Hazardous materials transportation is regulated by Title 49 of the code of federal regulations for the the global shipping community. The International Air Transport Association publishes the IATA Dangerous Goods Regulations manual. Develop Material Transfer Agreements for distribution of reagents and virus isolates and stocks to DAIDS supported investigators. Pick up incoming shipments from specific airport or other contract site of such deliveries to minimize inadvertent storage under less than optimal conditions and attend of reagent condition.

Agent Summary Statement is required for Human Immunodeficiency Viruses (HIVs) including HTLV-III, LAV, HIV-1 and HIV-2 and Occupationally Acquired Human Immunodeficiency Virus infections in Laboratories producing virus concentrates in large quantities.

A Report
Methods to Enhance Immune Responses to HIV
Developing Immune Responses
http://www.thebody.com/niaid/2004/hiv_vaccine.html

Says;
Immunogenicity refers to a vaccine or a component of a microorganism to stimulate immune responses and the two main types of immune responses are humoral and cellular immunity. Humoral immunity refers to protection provided by antibodies of the secreted products of one type of white blood cell called a B lymphocyte. Antibodies are custom-made proteins that circulate in body fluids (primarily blood and lymph) and specifically recognize foreign bacterial or viral components. Blymphocytes produce antibodies in response to a specific foreign invader like HIV or a vaccine.

Providing vaccines to generate more robust and long-lasting T cell response is important for both humoral and cell-mediated immunity. An effective way to enhance immune responses to HIV is to combine vaccines. Researchers first prepare or prime the immune systems of volunteers with one vaccine, such as a live vector vaccine (a bacterium or virus genetically engineered to contain a synthetic HIV gene) and then boost these responses with a different vaccine.

The Report titled -
Immune System Activation Boosts HIV Replication in HIV-Infected People
http://www.niaid.nih.gov/publications/agenda/0696/page3.htm

Says;
The normal activation of the immune system in response to microbes results in a transient increase in HIV replication, a phenom-

enon the NIH feels is important to the pathogenesis of HIV disease. Chronic immune activation, or the cumulative effect of multiple episodes of immune activation and bursts of virus production, probably contribute to the progression of HIV disease. Interestingly, the patients with the strongest immune systems had the largest increases in virus. This underscores the diabolical nature of HIV: the normal efforts of the immune system to mobilize itself and fight an invader results in HIV being revved up as well with a stronger immune system paradoxically leading to more viral replication. The researchers also examined immune system cells of the uninfected volunteers.

They found that cells from seven of these 10 people were more easily infected with HIV in the test tube after immunization than before immunization. In addition, the researchers found that cells from an uninfected subject became highly susceptible to HIV infection during an acute respiratory tract illness. Taken together with previous studies, our data suggest that ongoing immune activation may play a part in HIV pathogenesis, and may also enhance the susceptibility of uninfected people to HIV Drugs that could be used at certain times to dampen immune activation may also have a role in the treatment of HIV-infected people.Immune responses to persistent infections also may leave people more vulnerable to HIV infection.

A Report Titled -
August 2004 Special DAIDS Council Review
http://www.niaid.nih.gov/ncn/budget/concepts/c-aid0704.htm
Center for HIV/AIDS Vaccine Immunology (CHAVI)

Says;
CHAVI will support a systematic evaluation of vaccine candidates and immunization strategies that enhance potency, antigen presentation and immunogenicity, with a focus on novel adjuvants, particularly molecular adjuvants with potential for augmenting memory immune responses, and/or on approaches that induce persistent mucosal immune responses.

The overall goals of CHAVI will also include the systematic design and evaluation of immunogens and adjuvants eliciting persistent mucosal and/or systemic immune responses that can be explored in animal models and human studies.

An HIV/Anthrax based vaccine described at the International Aids Vaccine Initiative website located at www.iavi.org under the side heading of IAVI Database of AIDS Vaccines in Human Trial then search for all vaccines ever tested and the company is AVANT Immunotherapeutics, Inc. And the name of the vaccine is Lfn-p24

Says;

The WRAIR HIV vaccine designated LFn-p24 consists of an anthrax derived polypeptide called Lethal factor from which the toxin domain has been removed is fused to the HIV-1 gag p24 protein. The vaccine is aimed at inducing strong and persistent HIV-1 gag specific CD8 T Cell responses.

The NIAID HIV Vaccine glossary definition of seroconversion
http://www.niaid.nih.gov/factsheets/glossary.htm

Says;

seroconversion: the development of antibodies to a particular antigen. When people develop antibodies to HIV or an experimental HIV vaccine, they seroconvert from antibody-negative to antibody-positive. Vaccine-induced seroconversion does not represent an infection. Instead, vaccine-induced seroconversion is an expected response to vaccination that may disappear over time.

An FDA report
POINTS TO CONSIDER ON PLASMID DNA VACCINES FOR PREVENTIVE INFECTIOUS DISEASE INDICATIONS FOOD AND DRUG ADMINISTRATION Center for Biologics Evaluation and Research Office of Vaccine Research and Review
http://www.fda.gov/cber/gdlns/plasmid.txt
Genetic Toxicity
Says;

The effects of over expression of antigen from the DNA plasmid vaccine should also be considered. Aberrant expression of some proteins may lead to an inappropriate activation of the immune system, resulting in the generation of acute or chronic inflammatory responses, autoimmune sequelae, and destruction of normal tissues.

Where generation of an autoimmune response is potentially a risk in either the clinical trial or the preclinical testing, preclinical studies should be conducted over a long enough period to allow development of these disorders to appear.

The National Institute of Health Vaccine Glossary definition http://www.niaid.nih.gov/factsheets/glossary.htm autoimmunity: in HIV vaccination, a theoretical adverse effect in which the vaccine causes immune responses that are inappropriately directed at a person's own tissues.

A Report
Scientists Find HIV-Blocking Protein in Monkeys www.nih.gov/news/pr/feb2004/niaid-25.htm

Says;

NIAID is a component of the National Institutes of Health (NIH), an agency of the U.S. Department of Health and Human Services. NIAID supports basic and applied research such as HIV/AIDS, influenza, tuberculosis, malaria and illness from potential agents of bioterrorism. NIAID also supports research on transplantation and immune-related illnesses,including autoimmune disorders, asthma and allergies.

A Report
NIH AIDS Research Program Evaluation Vaccine Research & Development Area Review Panel Findings and Recommendations
http://www.nih.gov/od/oar/public/pubs/vaccine.pdf

Says;
The Clinical Trials program encompasses the NIAID-supported AVEG conducting evaluations of AIDS vaccine candidates designed

for baseline seroincidence information in high-risk cohorts and support for efficacy studies. Their are links to training and infrastructure for cohorts for epidemiological and intervention studies supported by the National Institute on Drug Abuse, and to studies on AIDS and sexually transmitted diseases at the Centers for Disease Control and Prevention. Together these sites and cohorts are adequate for the evaluation of vaccine candidates in humans.

(The report saying cohorts of individuals recruited at drug abuse centers and public health clinics are adequate for recruitment for the evaluation of vaccine candidates in humans is basically saying the so-called cohorts of people are along the lines of sub-human already being abused in cages. The intervention provided by the intentional lethal HIV clinical trials is for behavior modification for societal norms and status quotients in potions.

The only reason animals are being used is to cross-species infect humans. Targeting "cohorts" singled out for HIV clinical trials that affects everyone further exemplifies the discriminatory nature and hateful objectives the Bush Administration is infiltrating into the Vaccine Enterprise and into societal norms licensing to infect exclusively so-called "high risk" individuals that are allowed into the HIV clinical trials.)

The NIAID HIV Vaccine glossary definition of "cohort" located at http://www.niaid.nih.gov/factsheets/glossary.htm cohort: groups of individuals who share one or more characteristics in a research study and who are followed over time. For example, a vaccine trial might include two cohorts a group at low risk for HIV and a group at higher risk for HIV.

The National Institute of Health Vaccine Glossary definition of www.niaid.nih.gov/factsheets/glossary.htm intervention: a vaccine (or drug or "behavioral therapy") used in a clinical trial to improve health or alter the course of disease.

National Institutes
of Health
Fiscal Year 2001
Plan for HIV-Related
Research
PREPARED BY THE DIRECTOR
OFFICE OF AIDS RESEARCH
NATIONAL INSTITUTES OF HEALTH
www.nih.gov/od/oar/public/pubs/fy2001pln.pdf
Says;

With accumulating evidence in nonhuman primate studies and clinical studies that polyvalent antibodies can be effective for preventing transmission or altering disease course, it is timely to pursue the development of this strategy where prolonged or sustained intervention might be appropriate.

X: International
Research
www.nih.gov/od/oar/public/pubs/fy2006/10_international_fy2006.pdf
(search for "ramifications of HIV vaccines" at www.nih.gov)

Says;

Surveillance and epidemiologic studies indicate the epidemic continues to spread in both domestic and international settings. Reports of increases in risk behaviors and incidence of sexually transmitted diseases among men who have sex with men coupled with reports of high levels of seroprevalence among this population in major urban areas indicate the need for continued research on sexual behavior change. Because HIV-related behaviors, like all complex behaviors, are multiply determined. NIH research recognizes that no single approach to behavior change is going to be completely effective and much less so considering the varying populations that must be addressed. Therefore, the priorities call for greater involvement of all areas of behavioral and social science in identifying the contributions each can make. In addition, because HIV-related behaviors are governed by the same principles that govern all behavior the priorities call for greater leveraging of existing knowledge about behavioral principles to apply and test conclusions developed outside the field of HIV/AIDS research to addressing pressing problems of HIV/AIDS.

A Workshop Report
Rhesus Monkey Demands
in Biomedical Research
www.ncrr.nih.gov/compmed/rhesusworkshopreport.pdf

Says;

Researchers concluded that improving the efficiency of infection in the Indian rhesus model is an important goal. Dr. Shiu-Lok Hu of the Washington NPRC in Seattle intravenously administered SHIV KU-1 to immunized and "control" pigtailed macaques.

(The vaccine intervention using SHIV to immunize and control pigtailed macaques is what the Bush Administration is escalating in their newly forming Vaccine Enterprise infecting unprecedented numbers of innocent individuals to increase the number of controlled individuals, communities and nations to be under duress and certainly duress is not progress for a culturally diverse world of respect and dignity. The Bush Administration is aggressively trying to change society around the world to be easily controlled and defined sexually within a narrow minded scope of abstinence of energized individuality and starvation. Since Gays are seldom allowed to marry we are being singled out to be slowly destroyed by abstinence, and starvation along with behavior modification from the targeting strategies of the Bush Administration and co-sponsors of discrimination and death and dying. The disease equation of targeting "special populations" is being re-emerged similar to genocide in a Nazi type hate specialty of just another day evolving and nurturing judgement to equate to success of the Bush Administration. Human behavior being abused to succumb to be controlled is not living. Natural behavior is the only real aspect of the entire mess, and dissecting individuality with lab made diseases is pure evil selfishly denying the world of valuable expression towards peace. Love and expression are seldom found within the 21st century Bush Administration style republic and hence, their political force is maintaining destruction to paralyze and create fear in "others" because of the misuse of money and genetic engineering being used to exploit the immune system of "special populations" on many levels. And as a result, we are unable to live harmoniously always deciphering and being deciphered as a human product to keep or discard. We need desperately a concerted effort of reversing the man-made societal evolution leveraging health disparities as "novel" new decimating trends, designs and techniques that are propelling all aspects of health to decline at a virulent and alarming rate particularly in the targeted and "hardest hit" communities creating an adverse lopsided twilight zone affect destroying diversity of a spiritual nature of healthy transformation in love of nature on the ground and in the air.)

A Report
Factors Affecting Infectious Agent Pathogenicity
www.nih.gov
Says;

Nonhuman primates are not domesticated and as such carry viruses within their captive populations. New emerging infections are being discovered in baboons as recently evidenced by the discovery of a neuropathogenic reovirus. The notion that retroviruses and herpesviruses, have long fuses, and thus transmission may not become apparent for several years. Examples included HIV-1 and the AIDS epidemic which is generally considered to have arisen by cross-species transmission of SIVs to humans. Most commonly used methods to limit the spread of infectious diseases including barrier containment and quarantine for both the donor species and recipient are not likely to be effective for retroviruses since the use of quarantine is only useful for infectious disease where clinical signs are seen within the quarantine period.

(A monkey can be domesticated to enter a house thru a doggie door yet that does not mean the monkey will be behaviorally or politically correct once inside and as a result the monkey may be put into a cage in the basement of the politically incorrect house and abused years on end by the Bush Administration using viral intervention to control behavior abusing both humans and animals alike in depravity of human and animal communication being denied spiritual expression and injured by intervention. Domestication is discriminatory discipline in a cage the same as somebody's home or community deemed to be conducive for disease distribution to "hit hard" that debilitates the usage of appendages by way of immunization controlling pigtailed macaques as well as humans deemed lame excuses of nature being handicapped. Around and around the Bush Administration and co-sponsors of world control goes when they will stop terrorizing humanity nobody knows? Maybe reversed intervention to instruct the hate mongers on real domestication of caring and healing.

The human to nonhuman primate transmission is human researchers and scientists cross-infecting animal species to infect fellow humans in sterilized abstinence of humanized domesticated settings. The AIDS epidemic, which is generally considered to have arisen by cross-species transmission of SIVs is because of blood transfusions, injections and medicines using genetically engineered viruses fused together via laboratory technology and not sex as the public is led to believe as the cause of HIV disease. The garbage about nonhuman primates not being domesticated, and as a result carry viruses within their "captive populations" is hidden verbiage of a political nature of human "cohorts" deemed not domesticated adequately to the religious right to lives via standard operating domesticated Military procedures.

What is a captive population in the wild versus "domesticated" in a cage? Clinical settings are only insane distribution centers for disease and control while wild about living life in a community does not propagate disease as being centered and not controlled. Captive is domesticated and we are diseased on many levels of captivity to be brainwashed domesticated to open the flood gates of societal discrimination within ourselves and "others" as planned by the government and co-sponsors of wedging in disease distribution of violence to be further embedded in community under seige controlled and frustrated by laboratory disease.Behaviorally politically correct domestication is not likely to be effective for retroviruses until clinical signs of disease are seen within the quarantine period of political control propagating a catapult affect towards world control.

What is domesticated? Grooming? Hygiene adequate? Card carrying political asshole? It has to do with the government so-called evidenced based syndrome of illusion and making wild accusations that certain humans are better equipped as "fitter families" to control the world because of domestication is insane. The humans that are labeled nonprimate is insane accusations in a clinical caged setting to be abused or vice versus is reason for alarm today of all ear tagged in domestication cages to be intentionally neat and cleaned out by disease along the lines of sub-human already being abused in cages. The political lie that murders millions of animals of all shapes, sizes and colors is the worst domestication of the world to be uninhabitable getting worse everyday in societal pollution.

Captive populations and domestication means control by political humans misusing genetics and power to inhumanely alter our environment. The HIV/AIDS charade of "captive population" control by disease in America has primarily been Gay men, and until Gay men behave domestically, meaning abstinence without marriage or so-called Gay conversion enforcement, their will always be viruses around the corner to behaviorally challenge or stop us dead. The quarantine of Gays is still a political agenda on the back burner and these are life threatening and quality of life debilitating issues that still exist and haunt us today in evil domesticated America hitting us hard still labeling Gay a disease in a political clinical setting of the right winged hate mongers caged in their mental illnesses.

Even after more than two decades of people cashing in on death wrapped around a lie, many heterosexuals do realize the HIV/AIDS charade, yet the Bush Administration and co-sponsors punish people who stray away from their domesticated political window of quarantine. The political entrapment is only useful for infectious disease where clinical signs are seen within the quarantine period again exemplifies a political time frame of the Bush Administration and co-sponsors trying to gain absolute control obtaining more names and numbers for future contact attacks only if the political environment is more conducive for their entrenching infrastructure of domestication. Growing in numbers of American domestication of death and dying as status quo is sadly about grievance monied people already controlled to be dirty domesticated unnatural without a human care in the world. More sad is Americans afraid to talk for fear of being intrusively invaded and behaviorally modified again and again in past experiences learned and domesticated in harassing strategies of quarantine. Nobody should be proud to be an American infrastructure of domestication equating to decimation of friend as family. America is a dangerous environment to be controlled.

The misuse of money buying computer programs illustrating models of mutating populations evolving displaying a potential monetary windfall is not only a perilous business of mad science but bad leaders exploiting targeted populations to destroy and pollute nature. This combination is justification for impeachment of the current American bad and mad President G. Bush Jr. The world does not need this type of genetic superiority that lowers beauty to a second generation citizen . It is unnatural. Believe it or not there is room on this planet for everyone. The population dilemma is just another tired concept being embraced by tradition in order to divert the truth of American induced world control. Science has catapulted way beyond that nonsense and can preserve life with hybrid grains and food not destroy life with hybrid computer programs of deception, but yet again it is being held top secret by individuals only thinking of themselves. The HIV/AIDS agenda is being hidden in the vaults of nightmare generators of no minds of parallel universe of Karma and if they spent as much time on figuring out how to disperse the science in a positive manner, instead of calculating immune responses to pathogenic antigens and altering genes of targeted populations then there would be no world hunger for war. The living nightmare being sent from American labs will generate ill-will on this planet and bad memories for generations to come if this runaway train is not derailed. We are all better than that, so why not begin the transformation today? It would be a much more enjoyable adventure, instead of the current tired agendas that are painfully structured in venture capitalism.

The Bush Administration is using vaccines to intervene in behaviors of minority populations in all venues all across America. One example of the heinous and criminal actions and intent is a venue called the Broward House in Ft. Lauderdale, Fl. The Broward House has a website located at www.browardhouse.org and is a venue by which the Bush Administration is illegally mis-directing the uses of resources to target and control individuals with "inoculations," "re-inoculations," and "transference" in their so-called "risk for HIV and other issues" being the operative political motivator of "other issues" being control of a geographical location. Within The Broward House is a department called Intervention Broward which is a federally funded project whose purpose is to redirect and intervene in the lives of at-risk, substance abusing individuals from racial or ethnic minority groups who have recently been incarcerated. The intervention will take place through the provision of a comprehensive, personalized, intensive case management service delivery program."Intervention Broward" is a "intensive case management service delivery program with impairative aspects being "re-inoculation" and "transference."

Intervention Broward is a Bush Administration control strategy attempting to Bushwack and "hit hard" Broward county Florida. The targeting minorities political techniques with a virus vaccine is designed to further debilitate a community comprised of diversity already "hit hard" by HIV/AIDS. The inoculations and re-inoculations are designed to control and enable "transference" of feelings to a lifestyle of desparity feeling controlled by the Bush Administration and co-sponsors of their "high risk" behaviors. The virus vaccines are to control so-called behaviors thru declining health complications related to their vaccines taxing the community system already "hit hard". Intervention Broward is not a clinical trial, but the Bush Administration and co-sponsors have installed a dictating infrastructure for many other venues of viral distribution. It is still using lethal vaccines and medicines illegally anywhere and everywhere they have a venue such as The Broward House to claw their way into a community at risk of being targeted and slammed against the wall.)

The definition of inoculation per the Merriam Webster's Medical Desk Dictionary Revisied Edition is; a: the introduction of a microorganism into a medium suitable for its growth b: the introduction of a pathogen or antigen into a living organism to stimulate the production of antibodies.

The definition of transference per the Merriam Webster's Medical Desk Dictionary Revisied Edition is; transference : the redirection of feelings and desires and especially of those unconsciously retained from childhood toward a new object.

(The Bush Administration does not own anyone, and especially a person's feelings and desires to be transfered to transfer the life out of a person, and once viruses are inoculated or re-inoculated the choices not to be controlled by a set of circumstances that destroys joy are virtually non-existent. In addition, when an individuals life is intensely case managed, the Bush Administration's control over feelings and desires increases as well as manipulation of behavior. The feelings and desires the Bush Administration is attempting to transfer to a new object within the Vaccine Enterprise and the Broward House venue is not only in reference to drugs and jail, but also Gay feelings and desires. Adding substance abuse and jail intervention with HIV is the Bush Administration's attempts to redirect the public's feelings towards people with feelings and desires into segregation and discrimination. The Bush Administration's HIV/AIDS strategies are to redirect the focus that HIV is a behavioral issue and not their lethal vaccines and medicines.

The Bush Administration is leading the public to believe that HIV is somehow a mental behavioral issue and imprisonment, and once again stigmatizing HIV labeled a person, thus creating more hardships for all people living with HIV/AIDS. Jail time, substance abuse and HIV are not separate issues in the abuse category of government and industry abusing people with viral disease causing HIV drug usage and imprisonment. The Bush Administration is politically attempting to create and redirect public opinion into public outrage against certain labeled populations and in turn creates pathetic minds. The Bush Administration is a menace to society. Abusing each issue of jail time, substance abuse, and HIV by tossing each at each other in a collective melting pot of something HIV, jail time or substance abuse are not to gain a political momentum saying each issue are people is resulting in stigmatizing many more groups of people to say people are not worth a vote in who controls a life.The Bush Administration does not own people.

Forms of long term government torture to change America into a place of unhappiness and torture is because America is turning Militarily Globalized beginning with don't ask don't tell Silence = Death. Can anyone be happy in a country that tortures people with an infrastructure of inroads to join torture by bargaining for personal gain at the expense of others? The Bush Administration uses their torturous infrastructure for altruistic means.

The Bush Administration wants to stigmatize further the hidden truths regarding the HIV/AIDS charade to entrench an infrastructure with roots of evil. When someone goes to a cancer center they are not subjected to the same foggy and mis-directed federally funded crap, yet cancer is the same as AIDS. It is just another Bush Administration strategy to give the impression that people living with HIV/AIDS have additional issues and criminal behaviors, but the real fact is the criminal behaviors are with the bush administration.

The Broward House Intervention Broward department also has an extension program called CDC African American MSM (men who have sex with men) program. The website states the program targets African American gay men in the community who are at risk for HIV and other infectious diseases. The community is targeted through outreach, counseling, and testing, group level workshops and interventions, and one-on-one intervention services.

The CDC African American MSM (men who have sex with men) program is a program to control perceived behaviors thru targeting and infecting African American Gay Men. The Bush Administration perceives healthier living as a twisted set of ideals instead of the physical health of a person the same as the Bush Administration emphasizing and advertising quality of life meaning in their terms money, and since the inoculation and re-inoculation are health debilitating healthier living is the Bush Administration's destructive definition of the phrase with designs to basically control an individual into "behaving" by decimating his or her quality of life to even get out of bed. The Bush Administration has demanded and outlined as healthier living with a lethal inoculation that forces people to "behave" to enhance the money objectives in the evil government and industry objectives to increase their chances of a dirty money laundry quality of life.

Organized religion and faith based hate based bias along with government and Pharmaceutical industry on the front lines is far removed from love. We are lost yet found is a disorder of hate when we were never lost except for being led astray by evil government. Calmness before the storm means so many different things, but we are calm in the storm in order to survive. Collecting thoughts in a nation that has a leader with no mind is a futile attempt at being happy. The Bush Administration's blood is nasty and wants separation but the blood that binds is for everlasting. Get it? We are separated by politics and greed and the fear instilled by politics to satisfy a greedy government has forced us to put living life on a back burner and replace living with slavery. Being gay is a part of life and a part of living, but the hate lives to find a definition of Gay as unworthy and lost so separation by fear can turn us against one another alone. The fear factor the Bush Administration is embedding with disease and war causes a reaction in the community nuclear family whereby we are drawn within and never get a chance to reach out to each other.

I am gay, but the religious right says I am lost, and as a result, as all Gay men are in the same situation of "at risk" of health being jeopardized from being targeted with hate to lose yet more time in lives of we are not lost only separated from life. We need to collectively concentrate on helping each other then our love will spread. If we can not lean on each other in love then what is the point? Learning to help one another without money as a motivator is the prize. However, time is wasting and lives are being decimated by the sphere of influence that is held together by money gluing evil strategies of an inordinate amount of people re-originating out of the evil White House underground revolving door. We need to arise out of their hole of fear and control that destructs because even in the next few years the Bush Administration's strategies and agendas will create many years of disastrous affects. The hard facts can not be ignored because the technology and the strategies behind the technology being abused are designed to last long after there is a Bush Administration dictating America to be domesticated. And forget ever being free after they have embedded furthering their claws of death under the fabric of life of no choices where the evil pigs are only capable of sustaining themselves of more heartache and sorrow decimating life.

A Report
Towards Globalization with a Human Face: Implementation of the UN Global Compact Initiative at Novartis www.unglobalcompact.org/irj/servlet/prt/portal/prtroot/com.sapportals.km.docs/ungc_html_content/learning/Berlin/case_abstracts/cs_novaris.pdf

(this report can also be found at www.unglobalcompact.org and then search with the word "torture" and this as well as other reports pop up.)

Says:

Globalization can be seen as the latest stage in the development of capitalism.

For some, the liberated flow of capital, goods, services, and ideas opens up immense opportunities of employment, income, and wealth. For others, it fosters the relative, if not absolute, impoverishment of whole groups of countries and the majority of their inhabitants. A recent analysis from globalization opponents can be summarized as showing that globalization policies have contributed to increased poverty, greater inequality between and within nations, more widespread hunger, increased corporate concentration, reduced social services, and decreased power of labor vis-à-vis global corporations.

The presidential address report titled "Remarks by the President on Signing of H.R. 1298" - May 27,2003 located at www.aidsresponsibility.org/index.cfm where the president says:

George Bush Jr. says many religious and educational institutions are doing effective work on the front line of the AIDS crisis and he thanked all the faith-based and community activists and leaders who are at the meeting and share passion and desire to help people who suffer. George Bush Jr. continues saying efforts took place long before he arrived in Washington and the legislation he signed launches an emergency effort that will provide $15 billion over the next five years to fight AIDS abroad. It is the largest, single up front commitment in history for an international public health program involving a specific disease. George Bush Jr. continues saying in the face of preventable death and suffering, many have a moral duty to act, and many are acting. The nation of Uganda is pursuing a successful strategy of prevention, emphasizing abstinence and marital fidelity, as well as the responsible use of condoms to prevent HIV transmission. George Bush Jr. continues saying many will set up a broad and efficient network to deliver drugs to the farthest reaches of Africa and even by motorcycle, or bicycle. Many will renovate and, where necessary, build and equip clinics and laboratories and provide HIV testing throughout all regions of the targeted countries as well as support abstinence-based prevention education for young people in schools and churches and community centers.

(Add a bit of faith based religion on top of a foundation of hate with a bit of Ebola, SARS or SHIV plus whatever else sent from beyond to the front lines of the HIV/AIDS charade war hitting hard targeted individuals and communities wrapped around uncompassionate faith and the Bush Administration and company along with the "traditional" faith based outfits and nobody will not have to worry about tossing designated people out of church since they will be too sick to attend. The Bush Administration wants to control people by behavior intervention via disease to stop people from having sex to control populating the spirit of life. Where are the churches that do not "ask members to leave the congregation if they discover they are HIV-positive" and fight for God's members? Even the religions are ei-

44

ther controlled or hypocritical. Where is the army of God in the silent evil war of lab viruses and clinical outcomes of death and dying?

My lover and past friend died of disease and was stigmatized by the military because of his faith in Gay America. He was murdered an incrementally arduous death. Do not ask yourself to be yourself in church or in the military because it could be a death sentence since government and company are actively targeting minority communities, yet if voices are not heard then it is easier to be targeted. The military is in control of the minds and bodies of the enlisted and the military is branching out with the aid of certain industry giants to cripple humanity and thus control the minds and bodies outside the confines of enlistment.

My friend died a needless death as all people labeled with AIDS, but there are no bad memories because their souls are good. The realization of the HIV/AIDS nightmare creates vivid accounts of immoral traditional America raping life originating within the countless number of viral antigens being altered daily in labs, and that is not something anyone can rest easily dead or alive. Each day is a new nightmare of lives being lost in despicable ways and memory is constantly anew with this realization and never fades. Madness and Sadness evolving out of hate sending the "vulnerable" to the front lines of life to pay homage to the evil human creatures that always ask and never tell the truth even on their knees in church. Sub-groups, cohorts and "subjects" labeled offenders sent by petty generals and judges to the front lines of the HIV/AIDS charade to be administered a shot as a result of directives from the evil Bush administration and company's crumbling souls hanging above on rafters directing traffic around their untouchable human bodies dictating and never praying. Faith and security are a dichotomy and never the two shall truly meet in America and around the world since trust in God is virtually nonexistent in protecting the innocent and the vulnerable. Faith based religious conservative right to life hypocrisy converging in the madness of HIV/AIDS is sacrilegious and evil personified protecting religious and government leaders in bullet proof chariots of fire ablaze in hell. Why are the HIV/AIDS charade players faith based in fear and dripping in blood?)

A Report
HRSA Care ACTION: Providing HIV/AIDS Care In A Changing
Environment; Spirituality and Treatment of People Living With HIV
Disease www.hab.hrsa.gov/publications/february2002.htm

Says;

The way people living with HIV disease answer spiritual questions
has profound implications for both their physical health and their
health care providers. A growing body of research shows strong con-
nections between the way people define the "meaning" of their illness
and the strength of their immune systems and their ability to cope with
illness and loss and even the likelihood that they will adhere to medical
treatment as prescribed.

Evidence increasingly suggests that the attitude of medical caregiv-
ers toward their patients' spirituality has serious ramifications for the
level of trust and cooperation between patient and provider and even
the efficacy of medical care itself. When someone says they don't have
time for a sexual or spiritual history, it may be because they are un-
comfortable or feel it's personal and intrusive. How else can anyone to
account for the surveys showing patients' willingness to discuss issues
like their sexual behavior or spirituality but only if their doctor brings
them up and the finding that a majority of patients have not discussed
such matters with their doctors?

(Profound implications for the health care providers on the way patients answer spiritual questions regarding HIV/AIDS is the underlying
infrastructure of death and dying. God is watching us and dependent
upon spirtuality questions answered the doctor patient relationship can
be good or bad with the underlying infrastructure of death and dying
being non-negotiable as the political infrastructure embedded. Serious
ramifications on medical care itself due to spiritual questions answered
is upside down awareness and love for God.)

A report
Interpretation and Use of the Western Blot Assay for Serodiagnosis
of Human Immunodeficiency Virus Type 1 Infections
www.cdc.gov/mmwr/preview/mmwrhtml/00001431.htm

Says;

Clinical diagnosis and follow-up of patients is the responsibility
of the clinical practitioner. Serologic test results are but one contribution to a patient's data base, which contains medical history (including
high-risk behavior or exposure to HIV), results of physical examina-
tion, and other clinical findings. Clinicians must consider the total
profile for a client when attempting to make a diagnosis after indeterminate Western blot results have been obtained. Accurate diagnosis for
such persons can be challenging--and the challenge can be complicated
by the tendency of some clients to become distressed by the apparent
uncertainty of their test results.

Clinical follow-up of patients with indeterminate Western blot
results may require many months of observation, interviewing, and
testing.

A report titled:
HIV Infection and AIDS, An Overview
National Institutes of Health, National Institute for Allergy and
Infectious Disease - May 2000

Says;

Doctors diagnose HIV infection by using two different types of
antibody tests, ELISA and Western Blot. If a person is highly likely
to be infected with HIV and yet both tests are negative, a doctor may
look for HIV itself in the blood. The person also may be told to repeat
antibody testing at a later date, when antibodies to HIV are more likely
to have developed.

(If a person is highly likely to be infected with HIV and yet both tests are negative, a doctor may look for HIV itself in the blood and then the person may be told to repeat antibody testing at a later date, when antibodies to HIV are more likely to have developed illustrates the intentional infections taking place by unscrupulous doctors looking for HIV itself in the blood. If a person is highly likely to be infected with HIV yet both tests are negative yet the doctor looks for HIV in the blood is not only discriminating and unethical, but the aggressive government and company associated doctor desperate to find HIV in a person labeled "highly likely" or "high risk" inserts a virus and told to repeat antibody testing at a later date when antibodies to HIV are more likely to have developed. The doctor while searching for antibodies to HIV when both tests were negative is an intentional insertion of a virus (reagent) and then told to return at a later date so the HIV tests will show HIV positive is the sad reality behind the HIV/AIDS charade being allowed to continue to propagate ignorance and hatred.)

A report
HIV/AIDS, Sexually Transmitted Diseases, and Tuberculosis Prevention News Update   July 11, 2002
CDC News Updates
Medical News
Hope for AIDS Vaccine Fades; News of Superinfection Case
www.thebody.com

Says;

Harvard Medical School's Dr. Bruce Walker startled scientists with an unusual case of a patient who despite building up an immune response to HIV acquired a second HIV infection from a closely related virus and suffered a major setback. Scientists could be heard cursing and gasping.

Over two years Walker treated 14 patients with HIV drugs immediately after infection for a few weeks and then took them off the medicine to allow their immune systems a chance to detect the viruses as they surged out of hiding. One of those patients, a gay Boston man, went through two rounds of on/off medication and seemed to be doing extraordinarily well. But within one month time the virus's replication surged and when genetically analyzed proved to be 12 percent different from the type of HIV in the patient just 30 days earlier. The patient's immune system was suddenly helpless. He never got a new response against the second virus and he declined clinically.

(The HIV drugs given and then stopped to allow their immune systems a chance to detect the viruses as they surged out of hiding is saying the HIV drugs (similar to the Doctor detailed that planted a virus in someone labeled "high risk" and then told the individual to return a few weeks later after the body had developed antibodies to the virus) infected the patient, but the Boston Gay man's immune system did not respond to the crap Dr. Walker administered to him because it drained his immune system completely and as a result the Boston Gay man's immune system shut down from the consequences of the lab generated superinfection leaving the man gasping unable to curse.)

A Report
Harvard Vaccine Team Exposes Potential Dark Side of Reliance on Cellular Immune Protection
http://www.thebody.com/tag/jan_feb02/ctl.html

Says -

Interviewed in a Mark Schoofs Wall Street Journal piece primate researcher David Watkins raises the specter of escape mutations occurring in vaccinated humans and being transmitted onwards potentially leading to the emergence of a supervirus. In addition the potential effects of vaccines that ameliorate disease but do not prevent infection found that under some circumstances scientists and researchers could potentially select for pathogens with increased virulence. Views of Watkins illustrate the theoretical basis for an increasing opposing views of opinion among HIV vaccine researchers. On one side there is a cadre displaying considerable enthusiasm and optimism about prospects for T-cell based vaccines, including Norm Letvin and the U.K.'s Andrew Mc Michael. However an increasing vocal group including Watkins but perhaps most often associated with Harvard primatologist Ron Desrosiers argues for caution and even going so far as to characterize the current mood of optimism over new vaccines as irresponsible.

Somewhere in the middle stoic realists such as antibody expert John Moore from Cornell acknowledge that T-cell-based vaccines are well worth testing, but expect that the addition of an effective antibody-based approach will be required to achieve truly protective immune responses.

The NIAID HIV Vaccine Glossary located at http://www.niaid.nih.gov/factsheets/glossary.htm definition of immunoglobulin: a general term for antibodies which bind to invading organisms leading to their destruction. There are five classes of immunoglobulins: IgA, IgG, IgM, IgD and IgE. (See also Antibody)

A NIH News Release
New Studies Offer Clues to AIDS Vaccine Design and Safety
http://www.nih.gov/news/pr/feb99/niaid-01.htm

Says;

None of the monkeys that had been passively immunized with neutralizing antibodies became infected with SHIV.

In another study conducted with scientists from the National Cancer Institute, Dr. Martin's research team investigated whether neutralizing antibodies to HIV can accelerate the removal of HIV from the blood of monkeys. The scientists measured HIV clearance after infusing large quantities of the virus into three groups of monkeys; animals that had been persistently infected with SHIV for several years, and therefore made antibodies that recognized the HIV proteins; uninfected animals that had received the anti-HIV antibodies as in the first study; and animals that has never been infected with HIV or SHIV. Researchers found that HIV rapidly disappeared from the blood in each group of animals, but in monkeys with neutralizing antibodies to HIV virus clearance occurred more than twice as fast as in animals lacking these antibodies.

(Everything is a lie in the HIV/AIDS charade and neutralizing antibodies can clear HIV from the body at 100% neutralization against known amounts of virus. The monkeys infused with neutralizing antibodies exhibited viral clearance and the lie is immune responses to viruses to create antibodies. Why not just an injection and/or medicine of antibodies to heal a sick and tired nation against a Military harms way? The truth is the antibodies and immunoglobins destroy antigens and achieve truly protective immune responses, yet the scheme of creating efforts to have the body create antibodies (via immune responses) when antibodies are readily available as the "cure" is ignorant. The preventative vaccination HIV agenda is a ploy to vaccinate vast numbers of so-called "high risk" negative individuals with debilitating viruses as a political agenda to cause harm to the disenfranchised. The new American wave is a combination of evil political and corporate entities such as the Bush Administration, Pharmaceutical industry and the Bill and Melinda Gates Foundation opposing life and supporting a political force of power over the people at all costs.

The government has altered and collected specific antibodies (immunoglobins) to the same degree as genetically engineered antigens (viruses and bacteria), but rarely uses the antibodies that actually do something more by inactivating the foreign bacterial or viral components before infecting cells. In addition, genetically engineered viruses being used to create antibodies by immune stimulation can debilitate the antibodies themselves thus leaving the individual vulnerable to the viruses the antibodies are custom made not to bind with any antiviral effects.)

The Jordan Report
www.niaid.nih.gov/dmid/vaccines/jordan20/jordan20_2002.pdf

Says;

Another theory is that the early envelope vaccines were based on laboratory strains of HIV. Primary isolates of HIV, in contrast, have undergone minimal passage in fresh human peripheral mononuclear cells and are generally much less susceptible to neutralization by HIV antibodies.

To address this, NIAID-supported researchers engineered a molecule that in animals induced antibody responses that neutralize a broader range of laboratory-adapted strains and several primary isolates of HIV. Given the importance of inducing broadly reactive antibodies, this construct is now being developed further, and plans are underway to test it in clinical trials.

The NIAID HIV Vaccine Glossary located at
http://www.niaid.nih.gov/factsheets/glossary.htm definition of antigen: any substance that stimulates the immune system to produce antibodies.

Antigens are often foreign substances such as invading bacteria or viruses. (See also immunogen. antigenic-adj.)

A Report

The current Status of HIV-1 Vaccine Development, 2004: Recomendations for the Future by The NIAID AIDS Vaccine Research Working Group
www.niaid.nih.gov/daids/vaccine/pdf/AVRWG/finalreport.pdf

Says;

It is also the case that certain isolates and ENV-pseudotypes, even bona fide primary isolates, are atypically easy to neutralize. The use of neutralization-sensitive viruses in assays with a modest sensitivity increase, and the ability to accurately quantify minor increases in neutralization, have allowed some investigators to make the claim that "we can neutralize primary isolates" with sera raised against their own test antigen. Being able to neutralize selected primary isolates is certainly necessary, but not sufficient. As always, judgement has to be applied when interpreting the true meaning of some claims.

The National Institutes
of Health
Fiscal Year 2001
Plan for HIV-Related
Research
PREPARED BY THE DIRECTOR
OFFICE OF AIDS RESEARCH
NATIONAL INSTITUTES OF HEALTH
www.nih.gov/od/oar/public/pubs/fy2001pln.pdf

Develop and test new vaccine strategies, alone or in combination, to induce broad functional immune responses. both humoral and cellular, mucosal and systemic.against primary NSI, R5- using HIV isolates from all genetic clades.

Develop immunological reagents, improved methodologies, and assays to measure viral neutralization; explore the mechanisms of virus neutralization and the reason(s) for the relative difficulty to neutralize primary isolates.

(The potential effects of vaccines that mimic disease but do not prevent infection and found that under some circumstances they could potentially select for pathogens with increased virulence with the specter of such escape mutations occurring in vaccinated humans and being transmitted onwards, potentially leading to the emergence of a supervirus is the vaccine agenda for all vaccines the Bush Administration and co-sponsors in crime are generating in populations around the world trying to evidence base discrimination amongst various populations creating more anguishing pain along with dissent and violence. The vaccines causing infections resulting in disease period is cause for alarm and depending on the targeted population or individual the vaccine could be made to cause an increase in virulence resulting in a more virulent pain. The current mood of optimism over new vaccines as irresponsible is a gross understatement. The vaccines are not only irresponsible, but are being used as weapons of mass destruction to build upon the existing manmade prison of infectious disease and stigmatized high risk groups into the indefinite future. An effective antibody-based approach will be required to achieve truly protective immune responses is the cure the Bush Administration is withholding. When will the madness stop? Antibody expert John Moore from Cornell admitted that an effective antibody based approach is essentially necessary to achieve truly protective immune responses is basically the realm of the entire lie enveloping the HIV/AIDS charade where antibodies are being intentionally hidden for true elimination from the viral concoctions and instead using debilitating CD4 T-cell vaccines to create immune responses that create antibodies. The political ignorance of somewhere in the middle stoic realists are just a figment and loss of what humanity is by a political Bush monster system of filthy greed and power over souls inhumanly targeting individuals and communities labeled vulnerable to hit hard. It is so sad we build political pedestals to put inanimate human objects up against our own nature to live unhealthy in body and spirit. America breeds violence. Why are we being punished for political monsters harming us?)

The Report titled
The current Status of HIV-1 Vaccine Development, 2004: Recomendations for the Future by The NIAID AIDS Vaccine Research Working Group
www.niaid.nih.gov/daids/vaccine/pdf/AVRWG/finalreport.pdf

Says;

Formalize a database of newly transmitted HIV-1 full-length sequences for construction of subtype and group centralized sequences for antigenicity and immunogenicity studies and include the sequences of breakthrough isolates from all HIV-1 vaccine trials.

A report
Dateline NIAID, June 1996 Disarmed HIV Delivers Genes to Rat Neurons www.niaid.nih.gov/publications/dateline/full/0696.htm

Current gene therapy vectors can only transfer genes into cells undergoing active cell division, the process by which new cells are produced. Gene therapy in cells that divide rarely, if ever-such as brain,

muscle, liver, and blood precursor cells requires that the cells be removed from the patient, infected with the vector while growing in
culture, and reimplanted in the patient.

The NIAID HIV Vaccine Glossary located at http://www.niaid.
nih.gov/factsheets/glossary.htm definitions of immunogenicity: the
ability of an antigen or vaccine to stimulate immune responses.

antigen: any substance that stimulates the immune system to produce antibodies.

Antigens are often foreign substances such as invading bacteria or
viruses. (See also immunogen. antigenic-adj.)

A Report titled:
AIDS Vaccines for the World: Working Together to Accelerate Development and Delivery www.iavi.org/file.cfm?fid=394

Says;

In preparing for Phase III clinical trials there has to be an increasing understanding among communities that breakthrough infections
are likely to occur despite the prevention resources offered to the volunteers and there are a number of issues that need exploring in the
current context of HIV clinical trials.

In addition, in countries that do not have large experience with
vaccine trials, especially in Africa, there has been an effort to involve
people who have been doing other AIDS-related work and "re-tool"
their previous knowledge to deal with AIDS vaccines.

(Re-tooling of people's knowledge of a previous HIV/AIDS distribution system to deal with a swift use AIDS vaccines to swiftly cause
disease in HIV Clinical Trials is the agenda of the Bush Administration
and co-sponsors increasing viral disease onset. IAVI is the Bill and Melinda Gates Foundation of the International AIDS Vaccine Initiative as
a conduit and another venue to more swiftly distribute disease.)

The NIAID HIV Vaccine glossary definition of "breakthrough infection" located at http://www.niaid.nih.gov/factsheets/glossary.htm

breakthrough infection: an infection, which the vaccine is intended to prevent, that occurs in a volunteer during the course of a vaccine trial. Such an infection is caused by exposure to the infectious agent and may occur before or after the vaccine has taken effect or all doses have been given.

(The infection is caused by exposure to the infectious agent and may occur before or after the vaccine has taken effect or all doses have been given are the vaccinations inducing immune responses that create antibodies to the genetically engineered infectious agents that are altering humans to be different species to stigmatize, discriminate and destroy. The infectious agents with HIV tags are being administered in which the antibodies to the vaccine trigger an HIV positive test result and the HIV testing is just another trap to snare individuals into taking lethal drugs to further the control element of the human immune system vulnerability and to be subjected to compromise of the body and soul eliminating God out of the equation.)

A Report
National Institute for Health Fiscal Year 2001 Plan for HIV-Related Research www.nih.gov/od/oar/public/pubs/fy2001pln.pdf

Says;

Characterize the transmitted viral subtypes and changes that are occurring in proposed trial sites and evaluate the impact that genetic polymorphisms in different racial or ethnic backgrounds might have on receptor usage or immune responsiveness

The National Institutes
of Health Fiscal Year 2001
Plan for HIV-Related Research
PREPARED BY THE DIRECTOR OFFICE OF AIDS RE-
SEARCH
NATIONAL INSTITUTES OF HEALTH
www.nih.gov/od/oar/public/pubs/fy2001pln.pdf

Says;

Validate and enhance the efficiency of neuropsychological and neurologic tests performed in the context of clinical trials to identify those
tests most capable of determining treatment-related changes in different age and cultural groups.

Develop, incorporate, and validate functional neurologic and quality-of-life scales that are aimed at measuring the impact of the nervous
system complications of HIV infection in clinical trials.

Validate and develop functional neurologic and quality-of-life
scales aimed at measuring the impact of the nervous system complications of HIV infection in clinical trials.

The HIV/AIDS epidemic in the United States it becoming disturb-
ingly clear that minority populations bear a disproportionate burden of
HIV infection and AIDS.

The Report titled Plenery Discussion - Future Directions located
at www.nih.gov

Says;

The most serious although less likely is the potential to generate
a new epidemic by introducing nonhuman infectious agents into the
human population.

Presentation from the 2000 Emerging Infectious Diseases Conference in Atlanta, Georgia Epidemiology, Evolution, and Future of the HIV/AIDS Pandemic http://www.cdc.gov/ncidod/eid/vol7no3_supp/levin.htm

Says;

Mathematical models are used to address several questions concerning the epidemiologic and evolutionary future of HIV/AIDS in human populations and analysis suggests that when HIV first enters a human population, and for many years the epidemic is driven by early transmissions possibly occurring before donors have seroconverted to HIV-positive status. New HIV infections in a subpopulation (risk group) may decline or level off due to the saturation of the susceptible hosts rather than to evolution of the virus or to the efficacy of intervention, education, and public health measures. Evolution in humans for resistance to HIV infection or for the infection to engender a lower death rate will require thousands of years and will be achieved only after vast numbers of persons die of AIDS. Evolution is unlikely to increase the virulence of HIV.

The National Institute of Health Vaccine Glossary located at http://www.niaid.nih.gov/factsheets/glossary.htm definitions of statistical significance: the probability that an event or difference occurred as a result of the intervention (vaccine) rather than by chance alone. This probability is determined by using statistical tests to evaluate collected data. Guidelines for defining significance are chosen before data collection begins.

adverse event: in a clinical trial, an unwanted effect detected in participants. The term is used whether or not the effect can be attributed to the vaccine under the study.

incidence: the rate of occurrence of some event, such as the number of individuals who get a disease divided by a total given population per unit of time.

A Report
NIH AIDS Research Program Evaluation Vaccine Research & Development Area Review Panel Findings and Recommendations
http://www.nih.gov/od/oar/public/pubs/vaccine.pdf

Says;

NIH-funded research must become the primary "discovery engine" to power vaccine development by the commercial sector and/or, if needed, by the Federal Government. Without a strong stimulus from NIH that included much needed basic information, the waning private sector interest in HIV vaccine may vanish altogether.

(Nothing is real or meaningful under the Bush Administration dictatorship. The growing recognition that the National Institute of Health must be the primary "discovery engine" to power vaccine development because of much needed "basic information" for "responsibility" to stop HIV/AIDS is insane. The Bush Administration is driving lethal research forward towards the development of a vaccine with no intent on releasing the "cure" already available against HIV/AIDS. The Bush Administration is currently in charge to pave the way for thousands of years of pain and suffering as a future via disease distribution to achieve a goal of unprecedented political power only after vast numbers of persons die of disease. America is far from intelligent.)

A report titled: NIAID Awards $81 Million for HIV Vaccine Development http://www.nih.gov/news/pr/sep2003/niaid-29a.htm

Monday, September 29, 2003
Epimmune, Inc., San Diego, California

Says;

Colleagues at Epimmune, in collaboration with researchers at Bavarian-Nordic in Denmark want to develop an epitope-based HIV vaccine to be given in a prime/boost regimen and Epitopes are the small pieces of a foreign protein which immune system cells attach and allow them to recognize a pathogen as foreign.

Epitopes have been selected to induce immune responses in most of the world's population.

Merriam Webster's Medical Desk Dictionary Revisied Edition definitions of epitope: a molecular region on the surface of an antigen capable of eliciting an immune response and of combining with the specific antibody produced by such a response.

US Department of Health and Human Services, National Institute of Alergy and Infectious Diseases (NIAID)
RFP-NIH-NIAID-DAIDS-05-18
AIDS Research and Reference Reagent Program

www.niaid.nih.gov/contract/archive/RFP0518.pdf
AIDS Research and Reference Reagent Program
DAIDS 05-18

Says;

The purpose of this contract is to support the National Institutes of Health (NIH) AIDS Research and Reference Reagent Program in achieving its goal of providing critical research reagents and resources to the scientific community. An important rate limiting step in basic research is the identification and distribution of state-of-the-art reagents and technology.

Since its establishment in 1988 the ARP has evolved from a small bank of research materials to a unique and versatile worldwide resource of critical reagents not otherwise readily available to the HIV/AIDS research community. In 2002 the ARP contract was amended to provide reagents for biodefense research and other infectious diseases including transmissible spongiform encephalopathies. In addition to research reagents for HIV/AIDS the ARP has provided reagents for hepatitis C virus, anthrax and Severe Acute Respiratory Syndrome coronavirus research. The ARP acquires state-of-the-art reagents; produces these reagents, standardized panels, and protocols and then provides these reagents at minimal cost to qualified investigators throughout the world.

(America is the bioterrorist threat emerging within America and around the world today deliberately emerging diseases and oftentimes labeling the infections HIV/AIDS.

The Bush Administration and company are launching a global vaccine initiative directed by the administration and company with stepped-up resources and obscurities prioritized to mutate many generations of all our futures.)

A report titled;
The NIH Research Response to Emerging and Re-emerging Infectious Diseases: Implications for Global Health
  http://www.niaid.nih.gov/director/statements/emerging.htm

Says;

Emerging, re-emerging, and deliberately emerging diseases pose a global public health challenge. NIAID is the federal agency charged with the responsibility for conducting and coordinating basic and clinical research to cope with infectious disease and plays a major role in our national response to these serious global health issues.

A report titled:
HIV Vaccines and Your Immune System
March 2002
What Is a Preventive Vaccine
  http://www.thebody.com/pinf/vaccines.html

Says;

The way companies and researchers report therapeutic vaccine study results can be a little misleading and generally this is not intentional or deliberate.

A Report
Preparing Now To Assure Access AIDS Vaccines For The World located at the International AIDS Vaccine Initiative website at
www.iavi.org/pdf/accessblueprint.pdf

Says;

Swift worldwide vaccination of at-risk persons will require a massive amount of new vaccine. However typical production curve for vaccine makers is to start small and build capacity over time. A completely different way of doing business will be needed in the case of HIV/AIDS for swift vaccination of an enormous number of at-risk individuals.

A Report
Anthony S. Fauci, M.D.
The NIH Research Response to Emerging and Re-emerging Infectious Diseases and Implications for Global Health
www.niaid.nih.gov/director/statements/emerging.htm

Says;

Infectious diseases have afflicted humanity throughout history and will continue for the indefinite future. Moreover, the viruses, bacteria, and parasites that cause infectious diseases continually and dramatically change over time as new pathogens emerge and familiar ones re-emerge with either new properties or in unfamiliar settings. For example, since the Acquired Immunodeficiency Syndrome was first recognized in 1981, this emerging disease has spread relentlessly throughout the world and now threatens to surpass in total fatalities both the Black Death of the 14th century and the influenza pandemic of 1918-1919 two other emerging infections that each killed tens of millions of people. In the past five years alone there has been the appearance of the West Nile and monkeypox viruses in the United States and an unprecedented number of human infections with avian influenza viruses as well as the emergence of a new infectious disease Severe Acute Respiratory Syndrome (SARS). Finally, the anthrax bioterrorist attacks of 2001 confronted us with a disease resulting from the deliberate release of an infectious agent. Effective national and global responses to infectious disease threats, whether they are emerging, re-emerging, or deliberately introduced involve many different types of activities and many organizations. NIAID, a component of the National Institutes of Health (NIH), is the lead Federal agency for conducting, supporting, and coordinating research on infectious diseases. A second component specifies NIAID's several roles after the emergence of influenza viruses with pandemic potential in humans. Foremost among these is to help develop and produce and clinically test vaccines at different doses and in different populations in our vaccine clinical trial sites and would coordinate closely with the Centers for Disease Control and Prevention (CDC), FDA, and WHO to ensure that a effective vaccine is available to the public as soon as possible.

A Report;
Witnesses Appearing Before the
Senate Subcommittee on Labor, Health and Human Services, Education and Related Agencies Appropriations Global HIV/AIDS and Severe Acute Respiratory Syndrome (SARS)
http://www.niaid.nih.gov/director/congress/2003/sars_aids_040803.htm

Says;

The scientific advances realized during 55 years of NAID research have been applied to long-standing global health problems such as asthma, autoimmune diseases, diarrheal diseases, malaria, and tuberculosis, as well as to diseases and pathogens that have recently emerged or re-emerged. Examples of the latter include the acquired immunodeficiency syndrome (AIDS), highly virulent influenza viruses, West Nile virus, drug-resistant microbes, severe acute respiratory syndrome (SARS), and a new kind of emerging disease - one spread deliberately by bioterrorists. As has been the case with AIDS and other emerging health crises, the NIAID response to the threat of bioterrorism has been swift and comprehensive, resulting already in important progress both in basic science and in the development of biodefense counter-measures.

The NIAID biodefense research program is anchored in the tra-ditional NIH processes of basic biomedical research; concurrently, we are aggressively pursuing the goal of translating the findings of basic research into definable and quantifiable endpoints such as diagnostics, therapeutics, and vaccines. NIAID historically has sought to translate basic research findings into "real-world" interventions, as with the vac-cines noted above. Until now, however, the path to product develop-ment has not been central to our research strategy. The attacks of Sep-tember 11, 2001, and the subsequent anthrax incidents have compelled us to modify somewhat the way we do business, with an increased focus on translational research and product development. This applied research is based on the strongest possible foundation of fundamental knowledge of pathogenic microbes and the host immune response.

(However ugly the situation escalates the Bush Administration is oblivious in constructing new viral containment buildings. Containing time is ignorance amplified and the myriad of genetically engineered viral constructs being churned out in their laboratories at an alarming pace will never give peace of mind even to the perps. These contain-ment buildings will house some of the most lethal, virulent and con-tagious adapted live and attenuated viruses ever dreamed up and way more dangerous than Osama Bin Laden or the most heinous American serial killer named G. Bush untouchable and free. These viral manipu-lations are currently being tested on animals and "special populations" never to be in the wild.)

A Report
Of Monkeys and Men: AIDS Vaccine R&D at a Crossroads?
Located at
http://www.avac.org/lib/lib/libOACW13.htm

Says;

Neal Nathanson, a University of Pennsylvania microbiologist and former director of the federal government's Office of AIDS Research says in the absence of stronger scientific evidence showing that the current crop of HIV vaccine candidates might work, the push to establish large clinical trial networks to test these products in Phase III trials runs the risk of "creating a monster that has to be fed".

(Gay would not be a top priority of the political few if HIV/AIDS were not a charade and an agenda of great importance of demise that requires constant feeding of hate energy to recruit and advertise Gays as a disease in order to validate HIV/AIDS as a constant reminder advertised that Gays are vulnerable to hate crimes and extinction. Turning a blind eye or walking away from the devastation of laboratory HIV/AIDS is not a humane society and pays no mind to the itching in our hearts that is a matter to be Gay as person or somebody interested in saving trees in the forest or interested in spiritual alternatives of peace on earth where life as a human is of great importance for all of humanity willing to be educated in acceptance for the betterment of nature and a person of nature as society as a whole constant concern for our energy to love. And not a monster that has to be fed to eliminate life uneducating in Silence = Death creating more hate crimes that come out of nowhere. The years of poilitical infrastructure creating disease and war is now bubbling to the surface more people needing to be fed in the increasing infrastructure of Silence = Death with intent on escalating hate crimes and strategies in public reversed awreness and increasing advertising dollars spent on escalating widespread emerging disease complete with fear and underlying opportunities putting money and greed over human life. We need to stop the bleeding so the monsterous infrastructure will die as fast as it ends life. Imagine focusing on a picture of Silence = Death out of desire or necessity. Imagine poverty of what Silence = Death means to somebody that lives within the confines under the thumb rules of the right winged republic that refuses anyone the right to explain Silence = Death. Imagine silence as a way of life living in America of death and dying as a fear factory manipulating main stream media as the right winged conservative desires Silence = Death for personal gain or the number of humans today being property of the monster that has to be fed directed to be robotic slaves of the big business of death and dying subsequently endorsing hate crimes in the real world and then vicariously relayed into a frenzy on mainstream media news as worthy status quo. Silence = Death or the monster that has to be fed is not a "special right" to a life to die a slow arduous death of HIV/AIDS and/or the ramifications of HIV/AIDS awareness that does not "have" to be fed to the wolves of Federated America being Bushwacked by the Vaccine and Medicine Enterprise of viral war into arms and mouths. Why is it so difficult to understand the Bush Administration is a group of thugs and reversed vigilantes of no good energy for oil creating unspoken laws with violence that creates silence depleting our human resources?

More AIDS related deaths and infections during the Bush Administration than any other administration is not by chance, but because the monster that has to be fed is the Bush Administration and escalating infrastructure delivering and distributing more deadly viruses every day. Why is silence so difficult to diiscuss? Is not everyone tired of the void in our lives of more friends as family dying creating more memories on an AIDS quilt of life lost to HIV/AIDS and internalizing the new silent killer of laboratory disease that lingers latent and does not stop? Reality and the facts of the HIV/AIDS charde is many single lifetimes rolled into values of life dying at an unprecedented pace more important than anyone realizing value to the environment educated in buying a hybrid car or riding in a car pool as a twisted contribution of little or no substance to the big picture of valuing life is not to ignore many lives living with HIV/AIDS in a cesspool of infrastructure, economics and venture capitalism at the expense of "others". Shame on America being forgetful to the end as life does pass us bye.)

An article in Discover Magazine
Why is AIDS Worse in Africa?

Says;

The rate of infection in some parts of the continent is 100 times higher than in the United States, yet sexual activity is similar. Epidemiologists, forced to reconsider their theories of how the disease spreads, have come up with surprising new insights. By Helen Epstein Photography by Kristen Ashburn/Contact Press Images DISCOVER Vol. 25 No. 02 | February 2004 | Biology & Medicine Continues saying;

Botswana seems an unlikely place for an AIDS epidemic. Vast and underpopulated, it is largely free of the teeming slums, war zones, and inner-city drug cultures that epidemiologists say are typical niches for the human immunodeficiency virus. Botswana is an African paradise. Shortly after gaining its independence from Britain in 1966, large diamond reserves were discovered, and the economy has since grown faster—and for longer—than that of virtually any other nation in the world. Education is free, corruption is rare, crime rates are low, and the nation has never been at war. Citizens are loyal: A visitor quickly learns that even mild criticism of anything related to Botswana is considered impolite. Yet this country, with all these advantages, has the highest HIV-infection rate in the world.

(Botswana is about diamond reserves and setting up infrastructures so the Bush Administration and their base of greedy murderers can infiltrate entire countries by way of disease and eventually control governments and countries. Botswana is not immune to the administrations ring of corruption. The U.S. Government has been distributing disease for years and coercing Africans to participate in the clinical trials. This is just the beginning of the end if it continues.)

A Report
UN Sec'y-General says HIV/AIDS has a "devastating impact" on African food Production www.iavi.org/viewfile.cfm?fid=323

Says;

The devastating impact of HIV/AIDS on food production– with 7 million African farmers already dead – is only too obvious... Infection rates are rising among African women– who account for eight out of 10 of Africa's small farmers... AIDS is decimating the work force, killing the most skilled and productive members of society– the teachers, the civil servants, the doctors, the scientists.

A Report titled (molecular sequencing)
ICAAC, September 17-20 in Toronto
www.thebody.com/atn/349/icaac.html

Says;

We usually find the HIV/AIDS presentations less important in even-numbered years, when ICAAC competes with the International AIDS Conference.

The report titled;
The Global HIV/AIDS Vaccine Enterprise:
Scientific Strategic Plan
www.avac.org

Says;

More new HIV infections and AIDS deaths occurred in 2004 than in any prior year. A vaccine is critical for the control of the pandemic.

The Global HIV Vaccine Enterprise is an alliance of independent organizations committed to accelerating the development of a preventive HIV/AIDS vaccine based on a shared scientific plan. The enterprise will seek to engage the best researchers who are willing to work in a highly collaborative manner and to dedicate the majority of their efforts to solve the fundamental roadblocks in HIV vaccine development.

(The messages of deceit are painful reminders of lives lost in silent agony of the truth hidden and unable to prevail. The Gay and Lesbian Community Center of South florida HIV/AIDS education section of their website for example located at http://www.glccftl.org/library/safer_sex/index.htm says "This site contains HIV prevention messages that may not be appropriate for all audiences. Since HIV infection is spread primarily through sexual practices or by sharing needles, prevention messages and programs may address these topics. If you are not seeking such information or may be offended by such materials, please exit this web site."

(How much more can we endure? The agendas of publicizing messages that say the concept of a human behavior is inappropriate and results in disease and saying the disease is a topic of offensiveness is a double edged sword that cuts deep into the hearts of the afflicted, but that is the agenda equating homosexuality and other labeled "subpopulations" with disease and perversion. Old time psychology tried the same thing, but was denounced, as will the new old time religious zealots with conservative rights of delusional superiority attitudes immersed and mutating sick minded science that has destroyed countless lives and disabled even more with publicized puzzling perceptions, concepts, messages and pious attitudes.)

A Report titled;
HIV & Civil Rights
A Report from the Frontlines of the HIV/AIDS Epidemic
NEW YORK – The American Civil Liberties Union today released a survey, HIV & Civil Rights: A Report from the Frontlines of the HIV/AIDS Epidemic, which details widespread civil rights violations throughout the U.S. against people with HIV/AIDS.
http://www.aclu.org/HIVAIDS/HIVAIDS.cfm?ID=14376&c=89

Meanwhile, the federal government is not focused on the epidemic spiraling out of control in poor communities of color or on how to protect young men who have sex with men. Instead, it is focused on preventing young people from learning the facts about HIV by concentrating funding in programs that teach only one message – abstinence until marriage.

Encouraging abstinence among young people may be a valuable way to build self-esteem and to promote emotional intimacy between young couples, but advocating abstinence until marriage is meaningless for gay and bisexual teenagers as long as same-sex couples are prohibited from marrying.

Many people avoid testing and treatment because they are terrified about the potential consequences of a breach of confidentiality: social stigma, rejection by loved ones, being evicted from an apartment, losing a job, and suffering harassment or violence. Because of that fear, more people get infected, more people get sick, and more people die.

Particularly in rural areas and in African American, Latino and Native American communities, people say that they are afraid of being abandoned by their families and rejected by their churches. In the Florida panhandle, some churches ask members to leave the congregation if they discover they are HIV-positive. Many people who use anonymous testing wait to access care because they are afraid to be put in the database. Even for people who are proactive in seeking medical care, the fear of social retribution and discrimination is so extreme that they are willing to travel from Alabama to Georgia to get tested or to drive 350 miles in Montana for treatment.

Breaches of confidentiality can and do unravel people's lives, forcing them to find new jobs, new schools, and new homes. Nearly every one of the providers interviewed reported serious violations of medical privacy."

Fear about unauthorized disclosure appears to be growing more acute now that most states require testing agencies to report the names of people who test positive or who seek treatment. Several CBOs expressed concern that people are avoiding testing and treatment specifically because of fear about the fact that the government keeps a list of people with HIV/AIDS. Public confidence in the local health department is damaged almost irreparably if people perceive a link between efforts to track the identities of people with HIV and efforts to prosecute people for transmission of HIV. (This truly is the most vial and grossly comprehensive living nightmare the world has seen. The recombination and genetic engineering of HIV, SARS, Ebola and Smallpox (Vaccinia) and other pathogens is beyond remorse. The bush administration wants to add to the worldwide partnership list of vaccine and drug devastation with an infrastructure of laboratories and Pharmaceutical companies combined within a facade of so-called "religious based" institutions being unaware, but yet "on the front lines" of the HIV/AIDS charade as a way of further hiding the continuum of hate and infection where compassion is abused by the scope of science of ignorance and hate to the point where some churches ask members to leave the congregation if they discover they are HIV-positive.

The biased "evidence-based" behavior studies the Bush Administration uses to justify their ill-hearted behavior of discrimination using genocide is sick. The behavior modeling and intervention by leveraging certain faith based ideals (i.e. heterosexual marriage and abstinence if not married) by using debilitating disease as the behavior intervention when marriage is not an option for many Gays does not even begin to compute, but witch hunt does compute to the targeting practices of the Bush Administration. The HIV/AIDS religious facade is a tragic agenda, and some religions are so disdainful that openly Gay is a burning cross inside un-welcomed in the house of their owned God manipulating themselves void of shame judging all the same.)

A report located at
www.niaid.nih.gov/newsroom/releases/phase3hiv.htm
Says;

NIAID will continue to support HIV research and development that is deemed relevant and supportive of the military mission. As a result of the January 4, 2002 shift of management the NIAID is now under the control of the Department of Defense and all HIV research and development must be deemed relevant and supportive of the military mission.

The CIPRA Report
http://www.niaid.nih.gov/daids/cipra/u01.htm under the heading Inclusion of Women and Minorities in Research Involving Human Subjects says; It is the policy of the NIH that women and members of minority groups and their sub-populations must be included in all NIH supported biomedical and behavioral research projects involving human subjects, unless a clear, compelling rationale, and justification are provided that inclusion is inappropriate with respect to the health of the subjects or the purpose of the research. This policy results from the NIH Revitalization Act of 1993. All investigators proposing research involving human subjects should read the UPDATED NIH Guidelines For Inclusion of Women and Minorities as Subjects in Clinical Research, published in the NIH Guide for Grants and Contracts on August 2, 2000 (http://grants.nih.gov/grants/guide/notice-files/NOT-OD-00-048.html); a complete copy of the updated Guidelines are available at: http://grants.nih.gov/grants/funding/women_min/guidelines_update.htm. The revisions relate to NIH-defined Phase III clinical trials and require: all applications or proposals and/or protocols to provide a description of plans to conduct analyses, as appropriate, to address differences by sex/gender and/or racial/ethnic groups, including subgroups if applicable and all investigators to report accrual, and to conduct and report analyses, as appropriate, by sex/gender and/or racial/ethnic group differences.

(This is taxpayer's money being used to attack immune systems with virtually all infectious agents since that is how the Bush Administration and company are irresponsibly conducting themselves by recruiting and segregating certain populations ear-tagged to receive virtually all infectious agents in discrete discrimination being distributed worldwide where minority populations and women already "must be included in all clinical trials", but yet an intensification in the recruiting and expanding of minority inclusion including new targets is cause for immediate alarm and should be terminated immediately.

The Bush Administration's UPDATED NIH Guidelines For Inclusion of Women and Minorities as Subjects in Clinical Research describes blatant and obvious discriminatory approaches that are dangerous on purpose to get closer to their agendas of creating a world of "subjects" as slaves including sacrificing life as mere human resources as slaves. The direction of the firm hand viruses are being used to obey future hypocritical leaders imprisoned in hate. The "Update" states that research is to target and address differences by sex/gender and/or racial/ethnic groups, including subgroups if applicable and all investigators to report accrual, and to conduct and report analyses, as appropriate, by sex/gender and/or racial/ethnic group differences. The update under the Bush Administration is a blatant attack on what the administration labels as under-served communities being intentionally disenfranchised, and thereby once again, using eloquent verbiage to entrap innocent individuals and hide the intentional destruction indicative of the Bush Administration intentionally undermining communities to dig for gold they believe are in potential "subjects" to serve as slaves and weed out the rest. The so-called "evidence based" biased analyzation and reporting on the differences of individuals is furthering the disparity amongst minorities both physically, as well as mentally, by entrenching ignorant governmental conveyances always submerged in a mentality of evil manipulation.

Instead of researching and searching for "evidenced based" differences to report in order to permanently isolate people why not search, research, analyze and report on the similarities and familiarities within all humans to eliminate the harmful consequences of discrimination and the future ramifications of a "subject" American caught in a nightmare of hierarchical stylized mentality to depress life?)

The NIH Vaccine Research Report
www.niaid.nih.gov/vrc/pdf/vrcsp.pdf

Develop a better understanding of the differences and similarities between the immune systems of people and nonhuman primates, so that information generated from the primate models can be confidently translated to strategies in humans.

(The Bush Administration and co-sponsors are terrorizing the streets of America propagating disease, discrimination and fear.

The Bush Administration is completely off base trying to conger up population based disease clonning and conning their way out of accountability by disease latency creating an infrastructure and environment of behaviors to disease to infect people then just walk away. Associating sexual behaviors with disease labeled HIV/AIDS is a lie as well as the insane reality being controlled by irresponsible pious government behaviors pointing fingers. advertising and publicizing a disease designed to blame the individual for societal woes of disease distribution. The Bush Administration and co-sponsors of disease distribution are pure evil with more time shifting towards more judgement to create more disparity while a disease harbors latently within an individual is ominously disgusting. Today under the Bush Administration is a sad political time destroying life by their building infrastructure of death and dying and no accountability. America is slowly shifting to a military culture wrought with corruption, torture and biased based bigotry garnering political tension as a ploy to divert the realities of HIV/AIDS the charade of disease and war. Time the Bush Administration and co-sponsors spend gathering "evidenced based" crap furthering along ignorance of upside down AIDS Awareness is wasting valuable time witnessing more people being abused and dying of disease.

The military intervention crap of don't ask don't tell mantra discussing cheerleading morale of sis boom bam more war against Silence = Death causing depression is a sad tactic being used by the Bush Administration and co-sponsors of war distributing viral weapons of mass destruction in a vial. Abusing tedious science to intervene against humans as behaviors to install silence is appalling. Calling upon publicity and disease as a hateful outwardly publicity stunt while Silence = Death rampages continuing as a good thing to not ask or tell anything but arrested if someone does not inform a sexual partner of HIV status is outrageously cruel American military behavior. However, typical of the right winged politicians supporting military war for personal monetary gains with plenty of blinders to distribute. Under the table viral distribution to get hate and ignorance into our lives is a lifestyle nobody should be proud to be an American. The Bush Administration and co-sponsors are full of nightmares living a military life of Riley conceptualizing what tainted male egos of superiority crap should be defined far from humanity. The billions of big business dollars being invested in HIV/AIDS harassment and disease initiatives built on lies destroying lives stemming out of hate for humanity by government and company behaviors that are 100% dangerous is tragic. Steeped in military egos America is being warped by tradition of war escalating into new and improved strategies advertised by delusions of the day. America is truly wasting away as a Nation and becoming a wasteland of buriel sites from sea to shining sea.

The HIV clinical trials are being planned to increase in numbers of humans being recruited by the thousands into each clinical trial and the Bush Administration and company are proud in bolstering their recruiting efforts to lie to deceitfully influence statistical human numbers considered to die off in time. The vaccines that induce custom made antibodies that do not recognize the invading bacteria or viruses of the antigen of interest being put into the vaccines is part of the HIV/AIDS charade that energizes the Bush Administration and company to create more disease and infections of a latency nature labeling people behaviors that are culturally publicized to be causation to societal disease.

The triggering of the latent virus installed into targeted individuals is as simple as infiltrating another genetically engineered antigen or medicine into the individual to activate the latent virus. The swift onset of disease mislabeled and stigmatized as AIDS directed at targeted individuals and communities and/or populations is an attack upon humanity wherever we live. The tens of thousands of HIV-1 sequences warehoused in labs and on databases for researchers to randomly pick and choose to deliver their disease of choice with HIV culturally sensitive ramifications to the spirit of mind and body is soulfully painful

75

and misaligned comprehensible. The slow burn of HIV/AIDS to make cultural copies of its self infecting innocent individuals with varying degrees of debilitating real life outcomes originating out of clinical sterility of insane killings will never fertilize humanity to grow and should at least be recognized as covered up. Latency affects taking place around the world daily is a disorder crippling our daily news. The death and dying machine of the Bush Administration and company with plans of controlling the world needs to be stopped on today's news to be on our stands for tomorrow.

The intentional and continued targeting of the gay community by government and the pharmaceutical industry has resulted in the gay community in America being realized as easy prey to abuse from an early age for America to grow up to be the "hardest hit community" in welcoming hate and discrimination. In addition, the targeted prisoners, injection drug useres and minority so-called "subpopulations" is an tradition of a continuum of layering and lumping and dividing to label in America to actively stigmatize as a learned behavior of laboratory virus violence hidden in discriminate outerwear is cruel and unusual punishment and torture.

HIV Infection in Minority Populations
http://www.niaid.nih.gov/factsheets/minor.htm

Says;

NIAID's AIDS research agenda includes conducting clinical trials that address the specific needs and concerns of minority populations, ensuring that minority patients have access to all clinical trials and to the latest information on AIDS treatment and prevention. Together, these programs represent the largest AIDS treatment and prevention initiative in the world. Recruiting minorities into clinical trials is a priority for NIAID to ensure that research results will apply to all populations affected by HIV. Racial and ethnic minority populations in the United States, primarily African Americans and Hispanics, constitute 61 percent of the more than 830,000 cases of AIDS reported to the

U.S. Centers for Disease Control and Prevention (CDC) since the epidemic began in 1981.

(Recruiting minorities into clinical trials is a priority for NIAID to ensure that research results will apply to all populations affected by HIV is indicative of the discriminatory presence of the Bush Administration and co-sponsors of death and dying abusing "minorities" to apply to all populations to interpret "minorities" adversely under results and people being manipulated and labeled.)

HIV Prevention Strategic Plan Through 2005 located at www.cdc. gov/hiv/pubs/prev-strat-plan.pdf says:

CDC estimates that 70% of all new infections are among men, with gay men accounting for the majority 60% of those infections

NIH HEALTH DISPARITIES STRATEGIC PLAN EXPECTED IN SIX MONTHS
By: Jonathan Radow,from WASHINGTON FAX - March 9, 2004
http://lgbthealth.net/archive04/weeklyupdates04_3.html

Says;

A summary provided by NCMHD notes one of the main ideas expressed in the comments is that NIH should "increase the numbers of health disparities populations studied" to include more frequently the lesbian, gay, bisexual and transgender communities, as well as prisoners and under represented ethnic subpopulations, such as Haitians or the Hmong.

For both the minority health and health disparities reports, the guidance refers to five categories: basic research, clinical research, infrastructure, research training and career development and outreach.

Criteria for each category differ. For example, basic research may be counted as pertaining to minority health only if it meets certain standards, one of which is to involve a disease, condition or biological process that affects exclusively or almost exclusively one or more minority populations.

Other recurrent themes are NIH should "use racially and culturally sensitive and appropriate communication," and the agency should expand the scope of scientific inquiry to include cultural, psychological, behavioral, social, racial and gender-based influences on health, as well as study different groups' access to health care.

Separately, the council endorsed the NIH Guidance on Minority Health and Health Disparities Research Definitions and Application Methodology" under assurances it could be altered if the definitions prove problematic down the road.

For the health disparities reports, ICs should include all activities that address issues with low socioeconomic status and rural populations plus those that are included in the minority health report.

(Main components of NIH, NIAID and the Vaccine and Medicine Enterprise, Recurrent themes are main components of their population targeting agendas. The NIH and the Bush Administration along with the co-sponsors of the Vaccine Enterprise agendas are to involve a disease, condition or biological process that affects exclusively or almost exclusively one or more minority populations with varying degrees of recruiting intensity dependant upon agenda and especially minority Gays of color to publicize blight and disparity.

The gay community has been particularly hit hard by government and industry targeting strategies to spread disease for years and now they want to more frequently attack the Gay community? When will it stop? The government and industry deceit continues saying the NIH should use racially and culturally sensitive and appropriate communication, and expand the scope of scientific inquiry to include cultural, psychological, behavioral, social, racial and gender-based influences on health, as well as study different groups' access to health care is insane designs and strategies of the NIH and the Vaccine and Medicine

Enterprise creating infrastructure to validate escalating infiltration of communities on larger more intrusive scales to create new forms of discrimination involving more and more frequently distributed diseases.

The access to health care within the Vaccine Enterprise infiltration with disease is a continuum of disasters being put into a scale of horror within the HIV clinical trials staging population based final episodes and adverse health outcomes with quality of life ramifications to be weaned onto pharmaceuticals and out into the real world is excruciatingly painful and arduous inclusive of societal pain and stigma. Evidence basing people to be advertised different in real life by a disease is awful being exited out of life by strategies of clinical trials to distribute upside down AIDS Awareness posters so thousands more can be abused in the vicious growing cycle of escalating viral distribution. HIV clinical trials are garbage in an end stage pill or a needle and a syringe to further manipulate society by propagating fear and mistrust. With more clinical trials on the horizon to include more tens of thousands of individuals is disgusting.)

National Institutes
of Health
Fiscal Year 2001
Plan for HIV-Related
Research
PREPARED BY THE DIRECTOR
OFFICE OF AIDS RESEARCH
NATIONAL INSTITUTES OF HEALTH
www.nih.gov/od/oar/public/pubs/fy2001pln.pdf

Says;

HIV/AIDS vaccine research requires trained health care, medical research, and prevention specialists from the populations at risk who will be integrally involved in development of vaccine candidates and clinical vaccine and prevention trials. Trial-related research must develop outreach and incorporate education to include at risk populations from disadvantaged settings. International and domestic trial sites also need to develop a cadre of trained indigenous or minority personnel for the interdisciplinary research needed for the conduct of vaccine trials so that there is direct involvement of communities in vaccine trials at all levels and that trials are conducted in a collaborative manner.

A Report
Reagent Resource Support for AIDS Vaccine Development
located at www.niaid.nih.gov/contract/archive/rfp0301.pdf

Says;

Use and update a record-keeping system verifying all investigators and institutions requesting agents or reagents are in compliance with the requirements of the USA Patriot Act, Sec. 817.– Expansion of Biological Weapons Statute http://uscis.gov/graphics/lawsregs/patriot.pdf.

Obtain the appropriate licenses and permits required by local, State and Federal authorities for the safe import, handling, storage and distribution of reagents and drugs. Obtain appropriate interstate, intrastate and foreign import/export shipping licenses and permits for transporting biohazardous, infectious, and/or radioactive reagents and drugs. Provide safe packaging, shipping and distribution of reagents and drugs to selected research investigators in the U.S. and abroad so that shipments are coordinated for timely receipt. A secure package tracking system must be utilized to ensure that all materials are delivered to the intended recipient.

A report titled Dateline NIAID, June 1996 Disarmed HIV Delivers Genes to Rat Neurons
www.niaid.nih.gov/publications/dateline/full/0696.htm

Says;

Dr. Trono and his colleague Inder Verma, Ph.D., who receives funding from the National Cancer Institute and the National Heart, Lung, and Blood Institute, constructed a retroviral vector composed of elements of HIV and two other viruses. Only those HIV genetic sequences that control integration into the target cells genome were included.

A Report titled Factors Which Restrict Post-Entry Stages of Pathogenesis www.nih.gov

Says;

Viral gene products interacting with human proteins could thus represent predictors of transmissibility.

(Viral gene products are predictors of transmissibility not sexual behaviors.)

The Report titled Factors Affecting Infectious Pathogenicity www.nih.gov says;

Just as HIV-1 was spread through blood transfusions, simian retroviruses are poised to be transmitted in similar manners, either sexually or blood transfusions. In cases where the infection is silent and not yet characterized identification of an infection generally requires evidence of disease. In the worst case scenario, this could happen several decades after the transplants.

(The cases where infection is silent such as HIV/AIDS prior to disease requires disease to characterize and identify a person. HIV testing is a trap to reel in innocent individuals into the heinous HIV system to be labeled, discriminated and isolated as well as sold decimating drugs with vicious side affects.)

A Report titled;
Panel Session I: Cross-Species Transmission – Species Specificity and Tropism Says;

Infections could result in pathology that manifests many years after the transplant and some may give rise to cancers.

The Report Titled:

The current Status of HIV-1 Vaccine Development, 2004: Reco-mendations for the Future by The NIAID AIDS Vaccine Research Working Group

www.niaid.nih.gov/daids/vaccine/pdf/AVRWG/finalreport.pdf

Although the majority of global HIV-1 infections are aquired through heterosexual contact, this mode of infection is inefficient and generally involves transmission of only a subset of viruses from amongst a complex quasispecies.

A Report Under Vaccines" titled Recombinant Vaccinia Virus Vaccines dated 6/9/2004 located at http.www.ncbi.nlm.nih.gov/books/bv.fcgi?rid=vacc.section.53 or www.ncbi.nlm.nih.gov

Recombinant vaccinia viruses provide a powerful means of dissecting the immune responses of humans and experimental animals to individual gene products of infectious agents.

A recombinant vaccinia virus expressing the rabies virus glycoprotein has been successfully administered in bait form in a wildlife vaccine in both the United States and Europe.

(The political nature of bait is used in the HIV/AIDS charade to trap targeted humans to be infected with lab disease and in bait form for animals vaccinated with similar diseased bait to create similar unwanted fear of animals and needlessly eliminate animal friends as a "success".)

A Workshop Report
Rhesus Monkey Demands
in Biomedical Research
www.ncrr.nih.gov/compmed/rhesusworkshopreport.pdf

Says;

Develop new reagents and test new and existing reagents in alternative species.

The Resulting reagents and data will greatly enhance utility of alternative species for studies of infectious disease, immunology, genetics, and aging. Support research that expands basic knowledge about alternative species. Increase research on the natural biology, husbandry and veterinary care of alternative species particularly New World monkeys, which are less widely understood. Expertise must be developed and expanded in the husbandry and research uses of these species. This capacity building is best supported in laboratories where expertise currently exists with each of the species targeted for support. The opposite approach is to develop methodologies that can be used across monkey species, such as quantitative tests to measure viral RNA copies in plasma and immunological reagents for cell surface markers and cytokines. Dr. Keith Reimann of the New England NPRC has a Web site with information about commercially available immunological reagents that can be used across species. As scientists began exploring new concepts for preventing AIDS, the demand for macaques grew. The new field of microbicide research, for example, began to use the same macaque models as in vaccine research because the stocks for virus challenge were already titered for vaginal and rectal use in these animals.

The Report titled NIH AIDS Research Program Evaluation Vaccine Research & Development Area Review Panel Findings and Recommendations
http://www.nih.gov/od/oar/public/pubs/vaccine.pdf

The need for vaccines in human and veterinary medicine is now so obvious that the panel recommends the creation of a vaccine-dedicated study section.

(The only reason why vaccines are so obvious for humans and animals is the use of animals and humans in the labs to create cross-species adaptations of viruses once host range specific and many times do not cause disease in the natural host. The adaptations/recombinations (genetic engineering), however, has created a myriad of viruses that are pathogenic and being used to infect both animal and human via vaccines and drugs.)

The Report titled;
Panel Session I: Cross-Species Transmission – Species Specificity and Tropism http://www.niaid.nih.gov/dait/cross-species/page3.htm

Says;

Minor changes in some viruses can result in a change in tissue or species tropism. Coronaviruses (SARS) are particularly susceptioble to these events. In addition, one feline parvovirus changes into a canine parvovirus with relatively few nucleotide changes. FeLV-A, feline leukemia virus A, does not infect human cells, but it can undergo a few mutations and deletions to become FeLV-C and gain the ability to infect human cells. And in a pig parvovirus, a five amino acid mutation changes a nonpathogenic virus into one that is highly pathogenic.

And the gamma herpesviruses carry an IL-10 homologue, which switches the anti-viral, cytotoxic T helper 1 response to an antibody producing T helper 2 response. It has been observed that many large complex viruses have evolved genetic mechanisms for modulating immune responses that would otherwise attack them. Some of them carry genes that block tumor necrosis factor induction of infected cell apoptosis.

The Weekly News (TWN - South Florida's Gay Community Newspaper) December 9, 2004 issue under the heading Through Time states a Los Angeles Archbishop named Roger Mahoney as refuting the use of condoms to prevent AIDS saying Safe sex is both a lie and a fraud.

The Centers for Disease Control September 25, 1998 Morbidity And Mortality Weekly Report located at www.cdc.gov/mmwr/pdf/rr/rr4717.pdf says;

HIV can be transmitted efficiently through blood transfusions: an estimated 95% of recipients become infected from transfusion of a single unit of infected whole blood. The per-contact probability of transmission from an HIV- infected source is much lower for injecting-drug-use and sexual exposures. The risk for HIV transmission per episode of intravenous needle or syringe exposure is estimated at 0.67%. The risk per episode of percutaneous exposure (e.g., a needlestick) to HIV-infected blood is estimated at 0.4% (upper limit of 95% confidence interval [CI] = 0.8%) The risk for HIV transmission per episode of receptive penile-anal sexual exposure is estimated at 0.1%-3%; the risk per episode of receptive vaginal exposure is estimated at 0.1%-0.2%.

(Therefore, having receptive sex with an HIV Positive individual without the use of a condom is approximately 99.9% safe; the same as using a condom.)

The following reports illustrate further that HIV is not transmitted sexually; Failed to show risk for oral sex among 58,775 people receiving HIV counseling and tests. (California Dept. of Health Services, California HIV Testing & Counseling Quarterly Report, Office of AIDS/HIV Counsel. & Testing Section, July-September 1994.)

Receptive oral sex was not statistically significant for HIV sero-conversion. (Osmond, D., et al. HIV Infection in homosexual and bisexual men 18 to 29 years of age, American Journal of Public Health, 1994; 84:1933-7.)

No association could be demonstrated for any form of oral-genital contact. (Coates, R.A., et al. Risk factors for HIV infection in male sexual contacts of men with AIDS or AIDS-related condition," American Journal of Epidemiology, 1988; 128(4):729-39.)

The absence of detectable risk for seroconversion in the current study for oral genital intercourse is striking. (Kingsley, L.A., et al. Risk factors for seroconversion to human Immunodeficiency virus among male homosexuals, Lancet, 1987; 1(8529): 345-9.)

Our data suggest that HIV transmission through oral-genital contact is not very efficient. (Schaeker, Timothy, et al., Clinical and Epidemiologic Features of Primary HIV Infection, Annals of Internal Medicine, 1996; 125:257-264.)

There was no consistent evidence in the current study for oral-genital . . . transmission of HIV. (Moss, A., et al. "Risk factors for AIDS and HIV seropositivity, American Journal of Epidemiology, 1987; 125:1035-47.)

(There is no consistent evidence of oral genital...or genital genital transmission of HIV.)

The Report titled Of Monkeys and Men: AIDS Vaccine R&D at a Crossroads? Located at http://www.avac.org/lib/lib/libOACW13.htm

Says;

In another potential blow to AIDS vaccines based on cellular immunity to retard disease progression,   Bruce Walker and colleagues at Mass General reported that effective cellular immune responses didn't last very long among recently infected people who stopped their antiretroviral drugs after successfully suppressing the virus as part of so-called structured treatment interruptions.

Six months after the third treatment interruption, viral load began to rise and CD4 counts to drop among most of the individuals. But the study was small, involving only 14 people. A larger study will be needed to confirm the findings, the team reported.

A Report titled;
National Institute for Health Fiscal Year 2001 Plan for HIV-Related Research" located at
www.nih.gov/od/oar/public/pubs/fy2001pln.pdf

Says;

Mucosal immunity to viral and microbial antigens in animal and humans are being developed for optimal vaccine strategies of HIV antigen delivery. Live recombinant viral and bacterial vectors are being engineered to express one or more HIV proteins with attention to vectors that might provide dual benefit for HIV and some other pathogen. Vaccine vectors that target mucosal immune responses are being characterized for the potential negative side effects of candidate vaccine designs including the potential to increase the frequency of infection or the rate of disease progression in animal models.

(The Bush Administrations anti-sex agenda along with disease propagation is also being hidden in the concept of mucosal immunity which is fabricated terminology without any meaning except an additional avenue to distribute disease along with real life complications involving intentionally infecting targeted individuals and communities.)

A Report located at
http://www.thebody.com/niaid/2004/hiv_vaccine.html says;

HIV vaccines may also have to stimulate immunity at the mucous membranes that line the rectal and genital tract and induce what is called mucosal immunity.

A Workshop Report
"Rhesus Monkey Demands
in Biomedical Research"
www.ncrr.nih.gov/compmed/rhesusworkshopreport.pdf

As scientists began exploring new concepts for preventing AIDS, the demand for macaques grew. The new field of microbicide research, for example, began to use the same macaque models as in vaccine research because the stocks for virus challenge were already titered for vaginal and rectal use in these animals.

The NIH Vaccine research report located at
www.niaid.nih.gov/vrc/pdf/vrcsp.pdf

Says;

Technologies are being developed to evaluate mucosal cellular and humoral immune responses in macques as well as viral isolates that will allow reproducible mucosal SHIV/HIV virus challenges.

(The so-called mucosal immune system is being assaulted with the same crap as the so-called humoral and cellular immune systems yet not only with vaccines and medicines but with gels and topicals called microbicides. The gels and topicals are laced with bacteria, chemicals and viruses intended to be used during sex to spread disease the same as the vaccines and drugs in clinical settings.)

A Report
NIH AIDS Research Program Evaluation Vaccine Research & Development Area Review Panel Findings and Recommendations
http://www.nih.gov/od/oar/public/pubs/vaccine.pdf

Says;

Particular importance are studies concerning the basic immunology of the female and male genital tracts and exploration of effective immunization routes.

The Report titled
"CDC-FUNDED STUDY TO EXAMINE CRITICAL QUESTIONS IN HIV VACCINE RESEARCH April 2001"
www.cdc.gov/hiv/vaccine/vislaunchupd-3-30-2.pdf

Says;

Researchers are working with two of the six sites to investigate whether the vaccine produces a measurable antibody response at points of sexual exposure, including the penis, vagina and mouth, a response known as mucosal immunity.

The Microbicide Quality Assurance Program
http://www.mqap.org/projects.aspx

Says;

Scientists are evaluating the influence of the cell line in which the herpesvirus is grown and the project will be distributing herpesviruses grown in human and African green monkey cells to participating laboratories to be tested in their various microbicide assays.

The National Institutes of Health Fiscal Year 2003 Plan For HIV-Related Research www.oar.nih.gov/public/pubs/fy2003/iii_etiology.pdf

Says;

Scientific studies of AIDS related Kaposis Sarcoma have highlighted the potential causative role of a newly discovered human herpes virus HHV-8 angiogenic growth factors and HIV proteins released in the milieu of the etiology of this neoplasm.

A report titled;

Development of Topical Microbicides for Prevention of Human Immunodeficiency Virus and Herpes Simplex Virus Publisher: Blackwell Publishing

Says;

Vaginal inflammatory responses to topical microbicides may increase acquisition of HIV by several mechanisms. Proinflammatory cytokines may activate T-cells or macrophages rendering them more susceptible to HIV infection or in the case of HIV-infected individuals may induce viral replication in the reservoir of latently infected T-cells. Activation of HIV in latently infected cells up-regulate viral transcription in the vaginal mucosa and may accelerate the course of HIV infection or increase the risk of transmission.

Presently marketed topical microbicides are toxic and damage the vaginal epithelium with frequent use.Monitoring for cervicovaginal lesions by coloscopy has been routine during clinical microbicide clinical trials yet little is known about the more subtle changes in the cervicovaginal mucosal barrier including induction of mucosal inflamation and interference with host defense mechanisms.

(Presently marketed topical microbicides as well as the microbicides in clinical trials are cytotoxic and damage the vaginal epithelium with frequent use means that the currently marketed lubricants and lubricated condoms are toxic to human cells and induce mucosal inflamations and interference with host defense mechanisms as planned to intentionally infect cells rendering an individuals immune system defenseless with frequent use of the microbicides. It is the same nightmare as the vaccines and medicines touting prevention or behind the scenes abstinence for behavior and population control. Lubricants and lubricated condoms are marketed as preventative measures and advertised as protection yet that is a lie in the environment today of upside own security. The frequent use of microbicides increases the chance of up-regulation of viral transcription causing inflammation and infection caused by the viral ingredients in the microbicides expanding the vaccine and drug concepts contrived out of spite and anger. The administration is filled with ex-patriots performing acts of cruelty.)

An article
PROGRESS ON CALL TO DISCONTINUE NONOXYNOL-9 FOR RECTAL USE AND NEXT STEPS located at
      http://lgbthealth.net/archive04/weeklyupdates04_3.html says;

Durex Consumer Products announced in January that as of March 31, 2004 it will become the first of the three largest condom manufacturers to stop offering spermicidally lubricated condoms for sale and distribution. However the other two large condom manufacturers Ansell Ltd. maker of Lifestyles condoms and Church & Dwight Company maker of Trojan are still refusing to discontinue production of their N-9 condoms.

The report titled:
HIV Vaccines and Your Immune System
March 2002
http://www.thebody.com/pinf/vaccines.html

Says;

The process of recognizing a new critter such as an antigen or HIV and responding takes awhile. Also, if the way the particle of HIV was presented to the CD4+ cell was not done right, the entire process of antigen presentation, recognition and response could be crippled or ineffectual. Once a robust and effective response has been learned the immune system marshals full force against the "critter" to specifically contain and hopefully control or eliminate it entirely if possible.

A Report
How HIV Causes AIDS
EARLY EVENTS IN HIV INFECTION
http://www.niaid.nih.gov/factsheets/howhiv.htm

Says;

One reason that HIV is unique is the fact that despite the body's aggressive immune responses, which are sufficient to clear most viral infections, some HIV invariably escapes and it is due in large part to the high rate of mutations that occur during the process of HIV replication. Even when the virus does not avoid the immune system by mutating certain subsets of killer T cells that recognize HIV may be depleted or become dysfunctional.

A Report
CDC-FUNDED STUDY TO EXAMINE CRITICAL QUES-
TIONS IN HIV VACCINE RESEARCH April 2001
www.cdc.gov/hiv/vaccine/vislaunchupd-3-30-2.pdf

Says;

The vaccine seeks to elicit an immune response by introducing the body to the gp120 antigens, thereby producing antibodies that enable the immune system to clear HIV following exposure. If the vaccine is incapable of producing an antibody response sufficient to neutralize HIV, a secondary goal is to slow the natural course of HIV disease in those infected.

A Report
HIV Vaccines and Your Immune System
March 2002
http://www.thebody.com/pinf/vaccines.html

Says;

Still, researchers are exploring various strategies to improve HIV presentation and immune recognition and responses.

Studies showed that some products were more effective than others in inducing immune responses but it was wholly unclear if the responses had any impact in controlling HIV replication.

NIH News Release
New Studies Offer Clues to AIDS Vaccine Design and Safety
http://www.nih.gov/news/pr/feb99/niaid-01.htm

Says;

Defining the precise immune responses that a vaccine must induce to protect against infection with HIV will allow scientists to design tailor made vaccines that elicit those responses.

The National Institutes of Health Fiscal Year 2003 Plan For HIV-Related Research
www.oar.nih.gov/public/pubs/fy2003/iii_etiology.pdf

ETIOLOGY AND PATHOGENESIS
NIH Fiscal Year 2003 Plan for HIV-Related Research

Says;

HIV profoundly affects the immune system and as a result ongoing research is aimed at elucidating viraland immune mediated pathogenic processes resulting in the severe loss of immune function and inappropriate immune activation as well as disruption of immunomodulatory cytokine production and regulation observed in HIV infection and disease.

A Report titled "Merck Vaccine Studies for HIV"
www.atdn.org/trs/bull/bulletin13.html

Says;

Merck studied their vaccine in a group of monkeys. One group of monkeys was given the vaccine, and then challenged with a very large dose of an especially strong HIV-like virus. Another group of monkeys - the control group - was only given a very large dose of the virus. Most of the monkeys who just got the virus quickly developed AIDS and died. Researchers don't know how long the vaccinated monkeys will stay healthy, but the results were promising enough that Merck began testing the vaccine in HIV-negative people.

A Clinical Trial
Phase I Study of APL 400-003, a Candidate HIV Vaccine, in Negative Volunteers www.clinicaltrials.gov/ct/show/nct00001538?order=1

Says;

A plasmid DNA vaccine encoding the env and rev genes of HIV-1 in HIV-negative volunteers.

The National Institutes of Health Fiscal Year 2003 Plan For HIV-Related Research www.oar.nih.gov/public/pubs/fy2003/iii_etiology.pdf
ETIOLOGY AND PATHOGENESIS
NIH Fiscal Year 2003 Plan for HIV-Related Research

Says;

HIV can persist in a latent reservoir of resting memory CD4 T cells that is established very early after infection and by continuously replicating at very low levels and even in the presence of antiretroviral therapies able to drive viral load below the limits of detection.

NIH National Center for Research Resources
www.ncrr.nih.gov/newspub/apr02rpt/stories6.asp
Stories of Discovery
Monkey Viruses and Human AIDS

Says;

The more researchers learned about the monkey syndrome, the more obvious it became that the human and simian disorders were strikingly similar.

The Merriam Webster's Medical Desk Dictionary definition of Primates: an order of eutherian mammals including humans, apes, monkeys, lemurs, and extinct related forms that are all thought to be derived from generalized arboreal ancestors and that are in general characterized by increasing perfection of binocular vision, specialization of the appendages for grasping and enlargement and differentiation of the brain.

A Workshop Report
Rhesus Monkey Demands in Biomedical Research
www.ncrr.nih.gov/compmed/rhesusworkshopreport.pdf

Says;

The Southwest baboon colony has been extensively pedigreed beginning in the 1970s making it an incomparable primate resource for
genetic research. The pedigrees include thousands of baboons. Baboon
chromosomes are remarkably similar to human chromosomes in their
genetic arrangement. With a few rearrangements, the baboon gene
map can be aligned chromosome-for-chromosome with the human
gene. Macaques and baboons became evolutionarily separated from
each other about 7 million years ago which is the same duration of
time that chimpanzees and humans have been evolving independently.
The DNA sequences of macaques and baboons are about 98-99 percent identical likewise chimp and human DNA sequences are 98-99
percent identical. In addition, the karyotypes of macaque and baboons
are identical and no chromosome rearrangements have occurred during the 7 million years the animals have independently evolved. Therefore there is no innate genetic reason for choosing a macaque over a
baboon for biomedical research. The opposite approach is to develop
methodologies that can be used across monkey species such as quantitative tests to measure viral RNA copies in plasma and immunological
reagents for cell surface markers and cytokines. Dr. Keith Reimann of
the New England NPRC has a Web site with information about commercially available immunological reagents that can be used across species. As scientists began exploring new concepts for preventing AIDS
the demand for macaques grew. The new field of microbicide research
began to use the same macaque models as in vaccine research because
the stocks for virus challenge were already titered for vaginal and rectal
use in these animals.

The Workshop Report
Rhesus Monkey Demands
in Biomedical Research
www.ncrr.nih.gov/compmed/rhesusworkshopreport.pdf

http://www.ncrr.nih.gov/compmed/rhesusworkshopreport.pdf

Says;

Once virus genes were identified, researchers developed candidate vaccines and began testing them in rhesus and other macaque species, including pigtailed and cynomolgus macaques. Lack of standardization in macaque species, virus stocks, and outcome measures made comparisons among models difficult. Scientists began calling for a single model system, particularly for vaccine research.

The opposite approach is to develop methodologies that can be used across monkey species, such as quantitative tests to measure viral RNA copies in plasma and immunological reagents for cell surface markers and cytokines. Dr. Keith Reimann of the New England NPRC has a Web site with information about commercially available immunological reagents that can be used across species.

A Report
RFP NIH-NIAID-DAIDS-01-05" "HIV/SIV Database and Analysis Unit www.niaid.nih.gov/contract/archive/RFP0105.pdf

Maintain a database for studies conducted at the DAIDS-sponsored Simian Vaccine Evaluation Units (SVEU). This database shall include all protocol information and data summaries of each study conducted. Data within this database shall only be provided to the Project Officer and their designees, and shall not be included in website or hard-copy compendia unless requested by the Project Officer." Design and maintain, on a continuous basis, Internet web sites or other State-of-the Art dissemination methods for the purpose of disseminating information contained within all of the AIDS databases (with the exception of the database for studies conducted at the DAIDS sponsored Simian Vaccine Evaluation Units.)

An NIH Report
Scientists Find HIV Blocking Protein in Monkeys
Says;

Because monkeys are not susceptible to the human version of AIDS, results of vaccine trials conducted on them are not directly applicable to humans.

The NIH Vaccine Research Report
www.niaid.nih.gov/vrc/pdf/vrcsp.pdf

Develop a better understanding of the differences and similarities between the immune systems of people and nonhuman primates, so that information generated from the primate models can be confidently translated to strategies in humans.

A Report
Positives for Positives Spring 2004, Number 29
Interview with Peggy Johnston, PHD. Vaccine and Prevention Research Program NIAID, National Institutes of Health, Bethesda, Maryland Says;

There needs to be continued animal studies to study immunogenicity of new designs and how to induce it. There also needs to be continued human testing, because as one of the vaccine developers once said; "My sly monkeys sometimes lie, but humans never lie".

A Workshop Report
Rhesus Monkey Demands in Biomedical Research

Says;

More lentivirus challenge studies should be conducted using alternative macaque models, including Chinese rhesus, cynomolgus and pigtailed macaques. Also, more challenge studies should be conducted with SHIV.

An NIH News Release titled;
New Studies Offer Clues to AIDS Vaccine Design and Safety
http://www.nih.gov/news/pr/feb99/niaid-01.htm

Says;

By taking parts of the HIV envelope and parts of the inner core of SIV researchers have engineered simian-human immunodeficiency viruses (SHIVs) that mimic HIV infection and can cause AIDS-like illnesses in macaque monkeys. The chimeric viruses allows researching the responses of the immune system to the vaccines.

Study titled SHIV transmission and susceptibility to re-exposure through social contact Following vaccination with an HIV synthetic peptide-cocktail: a case study www.blackwell-synergy.com

Says;

As SHIV does not exist under natural conditions there is no specific information regarding its transmission.

The Study
SHIV transmission and susceptibility to re-exposure through social contact Following vaccination with an HIV synthetic peptide-cocktail: a case study www.blackwell-synergy.com

Says;

Little information is available in the literature about the natural transmission of simian immunodeficiency virus (SIV) in monkeys.

A Report titled Factors Which Restrict Post-Entry Stages of Pathogenesis www.nih.gov Says;

Simian immunodeficiency virus (SIV) replicates at high levels in the blood of infected African green monkeys without causing any symptoms or disease. All naturally occurring SIVs fail to cause immunodeficiency in their natural host and it will be important to determine why cross-species transmission turns these viruses into potent pathogens.

NIH National Center for Research Resources
www.ncrr.nih.gov/newspub/apr02rpt/stories6.asp
Stories of Discovery
Monkey Viruses and Human AIDS
Says;

Knowledge gained from SIV research demonstrates the importance of studying diseases that arise spontaneously in animals.

The National Institute of Health Vaccine Glossary located at http://www.niaid.nih.gov/factsheets/glossary.htm definition of

SHIV: genetically engineered hybrid virus having an HIV envelope and an SIV core.

National Institutes of Health Fiscal Year 2001
Plan for HIV-Related Research
PREPARED BY THE DIRECTOR OFFICE OF AIDS RE-SEARCH
NATIONAL INSTITUTES OF HEALTH
www.nih.gov/od/oar/public/pubs/fy2001pln.pdf

Says;

NIH is Developing and defining the associated epitopes of HIV/SIV proteins for vaccine studies for continued development to exploit SHIV chimeric viruses with varying degrees of virulence to more closely reflect disease progression observed in HIV-infected people with genetic variations observed in worldwide HIV epidemics.

A report
Gene Therapy for HIV
www.thebody.com/pinf/jul04/gene_therapy.html#challenges
under the heading of Challenges says;

Many researchers believe that the most effective way to get a gene into a cell is by packaging it into a virus. Viruses that scientists use to deliver genes, called vectors, include the adeno-associated virus and maybe even crippled versions of HIV.

A Report
Human Genome Project Information
Gene Therapy
www.ornl.gov/sci/techresources/Human_Genome/medicine/gene-therapy.html
or www.ornl.gov or www.doegenomes.org

Says;

A carrier molecule called a vector must be used to deliver the therapeutic gene to the patient's target cells. Currently, the most common vector is a virus that has been genetically altered to carry human DNA.

Viruses have evolved a way of encapsulating and delivering their genes to human cells in a pathogenic manner.

A Report
Scientists Find HIV-Blocking Protein in Monkeys
www.nih.gov/news/pr/feb2004/niaid-25.htm

Says;

Over the years scientists have learned quite a bit about how HIV enters cells. However, the steps between virus entry and conversion of the viral RNA into DNA have been a black box.

A key preparatory step is the removal of the protective shell surrounding HIV's genetic material. This coat called the capsid must be removed before HIV can insert its genetic material into the host cell's DNA and begin to make copies of itself.

A Report
Human Genome Project Information
Gene Therapy
www.ornl.gov/sci/techresources/Human_Genome/medicine/ge-netherapy.html
  or www.ornl.gov or www.doegenomes.org

Says;

Some of the different types of viruses used as gene therapy vectors:

Adenoviruses are viruses with double-stranded DNA genomes that cause respiratory, intestinal, and eye infections in humans.

Adeno-associated viruses are small single-stranded DNA viruses that can insert their genetic material at a specific site on chromosome 19.

Herpes simplex viruses are double-stranded DNA viruses that infect a particular cell type, neurons.

Retroviruses are viruses that can create double-stranded DNA copies of their RNA genomes and these copies of its genome can be integrated into the chromosomes of host cells. Human Immunodeficiency Virus (HIV) is a retrovirus.

(The DNA or T-cell based vaccines that infuse viruses encoding HIV retroviruses(RNA) into the DNA of individuals is scary business since the viruses have been genetically altered to hide from the neutralizing antibodies once the viruses have triggered an immune response to enter and alter the human cell. In addition, the Bush Administration improving vaccines to generate more robust and long-lasting T cell response is infusing a faster and more robust onset of death and dying at an unprecedented pace.)

A Report

PROGRESS IN HIV VACCINE RESEARCH
www.blackwell-synergy.com

Says;

Unfortunately the safety concerns with using a live attenuated retrovirus for adults can cause AIDS in neonatal macaques.

The Merriam Websters Medical Desk Dictionary Definition of
Retrovirus located at http://www.merriam-webster.com retrovirus: any of a family (Retroviridae) of single-stranded RNA viruses (as HIV and the Rous sarcoma virus) that produce reverse transcriptase by means of which DNA is synthesized using their RNA as a template and incorporated into the genome of infected cells and that include numerous tumorigenic viruses called also RNA tumor virus

The NIAID HIV Vaccine Glossary definitions of http://www.niaid.nih.gov/factsheets/glossary.htm retrovirus: HIV and other viruses that carry their genetic material in the form of RNA rather than DNA and have the enzyme reverse transcriptase that can transcribe it into DNA. In most animals and plants, DNA is usually made into RNA, hence "retro" is used to indicate the opposite direction.

reverse transcriptase: the enzyme produced by HIV and other retroviruses that enables them to direct a cell to synthesize DNA from their viral RNA

RNA: a single-stranded molecule composed of chemical building blocks, similar to DNA. The RNA segments in cells represent copies of portions of the DNA sequences in the nucleus. RNA is the sole genetic material of retroviruses.

The Merriam-Webster's Medical Desk Dictionary definitions

RNA virus: a virus (as a paramyxovirus or a retrovirus) whose genome consists of RNA

RNA tumor virus: RETROVIRUS

A Report
National Institute for Health Fiscal Year 2001 Plan for HIV-Related Research www.nih.gov/od/oar/public/pubs/fy2001pln

Says;

Selection of viral antigens for the design of an HIV vaccine. Viral and microbial antigens in animal and humans to develop optimal vaccine strategies for HIV antigen delivery. Study the mechanism of action of vaccine adjuvants and enhanced modes of HIV and related lentivirus antigen presentation to induce different cytokine responses and carry out research in non-human primates and human vaccinees.

The Merriam Websters Medical Desk Dictionary Definition

lentivirus: any of a genus of retroviruses that cause slowly progressive often fatal animal diseases (as AIDS) - lentiviral

The NIH National Center for Research Resources
www.ncrr.nih.gov/newspub/apr02rpt/stories6.asp
Stories of Discovery
Monkey Viruses and Human AIDS

Says;

In 1980 no one knew what caused AIDS. Suspects ranged from a variety of viruses to a recreational drug known as poppers. Without knowing the causative agent it was impossible to study or diagnose the earliest stages of human infection. A lead came in 1983 when two teams of scientists independently isolated a new human retrovirus with a genome consisting of RNA rather than DNA from the tissues of AIDS patients.

A Report
National Institute for Health Fiscal Year 2001 Plan for HIV-Related Research located at www.nih.gov/od/oar/public/pubs/fy2001pln.pdf

Says;

Support the design, development, production, and testing of novel HIV/AIDS vaccine candidates for safety and their ability to elicit appropriate antiviral immune responses that may include but are not limited to: Virus-like particles containing one or more virus proteins, peptides, or antigens; Live, recombinant viral and bacterial vectors engineered to express one or more HIV proteins with attention to vectors that might provide dual benefit for HIV and some other pathogen or to vaccine vectors that target mucosal immune responses. In addition support DNA or RNA coding for viral proteins.

A Report
Panel Session II: Cross-Species Transmission Mechanisms of Pathogen Adaptation www.vrc.nih.gov/dait/cross-species/pages6.htm

Says;

When cross-species transmission does result in human infection the retroviral sequences integrate stably into the human genome and can persist long-term.

The NIAID Vaccine glossary definitions of DNA vaccine located at http://www.niaid.nih.gov/factsheets/glossary.htm
Says;

DNA vaccine (nucleic acid vaccine):

direct injection of a gene(s) coding for a specific antigenic protein(s), resulting in direct production of such antigen(s) within the vaccine recipient in order to trigger an appropriate immune response.

The International AIDS Vaccine Initiative glossary definition of DNA vaccine located in the 2002 Annual Progress Report at
www.iavi.org/viewpage.cfm?aid=34

Says;

DNA Vaccine - An experimental vaccine technology in which one or more genes coding for specific antigen(s) are directly injected into the body, where they hopefully produce antigen(s) in the recipient and trigger immune responses.

The International AIDS Vaccine Initiative glossary definition of replicon located in the 2002 Annual Progress Report at
www.iavi.org/viewpage.cfm?aid=34 is

replicon; a unit of DNA that contains an initiation point and a termination point and is capable of self-replication. See DNA vaccine.

AIDS Vaccines for the World: Working Together to Accelerate Development and Delivery www.iavi.org/file.cfm?fid=394

Says;

A different approach is based on alphavirus replicon particles from Semliki Forest Virus. Large-scale monkey challenge studies will be used to compare and prioritize these second generation candidates.

A Report
Progress IN HIV VACCINE RESEARCH
www.blackwell-synergy.com
Says;

Most recently it also has been demonstrated that a live attenuated SIV vaccines can form virulent recombinations following challenge with virulent virus. The most worrying fact remains the integration of HIV into host DNA, not only leading to the likelihood of lifelong persistence of the vaccine virus as well as carrying the risk of insertional mutagenesis.

The NIH National Center for Research Resources
www.ncrr.nih.gov/newspub/apr02rpt/stories6.asp
Stories of Discovery
Monkey Viruses and Human AIDS
Says;

Some SIV vaccines completely protect animals from even the most deadly variants of SIV. These vaccines are made of live but weakened (or attenuated) strains of SIV, in which one or more viral genes are deleted. Vaccinated animals have remained virus-free and healthy for years after complete viral challenge. Since even a weakened virus may cause disease when used as a vaccine a live attenuated AIDS vaccines may be deemed too risky for human use.

The Report titled
"The current Status of HIV-1 Vaccine Development, 2004: Re-comendations for the Future by The NIAID AIDS Vaccine Research Working Group"
www.niaid.nih.gov/daids/vaccine/pdf/AVRWG/finalreport.pdf

Says;

Consider a new effort to define the correlates of protection for nef-deleted attenuated SIV, these correlates are still ill-defined. Define the role for other HIV regulatory genes as vaccine components.

A Report
New Studies Offer Clues to AIDS Vaccine Design and Safety
www.nih.gov/news/pr/feb99/niaid-01.htm

Says;

Findings confirmed that this triply deleted SIV candidate vaccine retained its ability to cause AIDS.

The Report titled;
Panel Session I: Cross-Species Transmission – Species Specificity and Tropism
www.nih.gov
http://www.niaid.nih.gov/dait/cross-species/page3.htm

Says;

SIV/PBJ is another pathogenic SIV derived from sooty mangabey. PBJ contains a mutation in the nef gene that allows the virus to induce an acutely lethal gastrointestinal (GI) disease. Animals that survive the initial GI attack later develop AIDS.

A Report
www.nih.gov
says;

A second simian retrovirus that must be considered in the transplant setting is SFV, another virus with high rates of infection in adult baboons (99 percent). While no disease association is apparent it has been shown to infect humans and the long term consequences of transmission to humans is unknown.

A report titled;
VAX 2(3), April 2004
http://www.iavireport.org/VAX/VAXApril2004.asp
Making vaccines

Says;

Drugs are usually produced by combining a variety of chemical compounds. But vaccines are made using biological systems, meaning that living organisms are used to produce the vaccine. Vaccine developers take advantage of the fact that animal cells and bacteria produce many different substances as part of their normal functions, and adapt these capabilities to help make vaccines."

National Institutes of Health
Strategic Plan
Research Toward Development of an
Effective AIDS Vaccine
www.vrc.nih.gov/vrc/pdf/vrcsp.pdf

Says;

The current platform for DNA immunization is also likely to require modifications to improve gene expression and gene delivery. To date, the VRC has constructed numerous immunogens by inserting HIV cDNAs into relevant plasmids. Construction of these immunogens includes modification of the nucleotide sequence for optimizing protein expression. Mutagenesis to define alternative proteins with enhanced immunogenicity will also be explored.

A Report titled
New Studies Offer Clues to AIDS Vaccine Design and Safety
www.nih.gov/news/pr/feb99/niaid-01.htm
Says;

Some scientists believe that a live, attenuated HIV vaccine composed of virus rendered non-pathogenic by removal of one or more essential genes- could be the best way to stimulate broad-based immunity to HIV. Some scientists, however question whether concerns about the safety of using live, attenuated HIV vaccines can be adequately addressed.

The Report
NIH National Center for Research Resources
www.ncrr.nih.gov/newspub/apr02rpt/stories6.asp
Stories of Discovery
Monkey Viruses and Human AIDS

Says;

Scientists have also identified portions of additional viral proteins that are displayed on infected cells and might be used to further enhance potential AIDS vaccines.

Although tat is displayed on all SIV- and HIV-infected CD4 cells, a few viruses have mutant versions of tat, which allow them to escape the killer T-cell assault. Eventually, these mutant viruses are able to repopulate the animal's bloodstream and cause full-blown infection.

The Report
NIH National Center for Research Resources
www.ncrr.nih.gov/newspub/apr02rpt/stories6.asp
Stories of Discovery
Monkey Viruses and Human AIDS

Since even a weakened virus may cause disease when used as a vaccine, live attenuated AIDS vaccines may be deemed too risky for human use.

The Report titled
"The current Status of HIV-1 Vaccine Development, 2004: Recomendations for the Future by The NIAID AIDS Vaccine Research Working Group"
www.niaid.nih.gov/daids/vaccine/pdf/AVRWG/finalreport.pdf

Says;

Accelerate basic science studies into live vector development to better understand the issues of pre-existing immunity to current vectors being developed, and induce durable immune responses. For example, proof of concept studies should be preformed quickly in order to understand the role of preexisting immunity on utility of recombinant adenoviral vectors, Modified Vaccinia Ankara (MVA) and other vectors in the pipeline. Vectors should be specifically sought for which pre-existing immunity is not an issue, and that induced long-lived immunity with one or two immunizations.

A report
AIDS Vaccines for the World: Working Together to Accelerate Development and Delivery www.iavi.org/file.cfm?fid=394

Says;

John Shiver, Merck and Co. Inc., discussed candidate AIDS vaccines being developed by his company. Focusing on results from uninfected volunteers, Shiver reported that the DNA vaccine alone shows detectable but relatively low immunogenicity, with the best responses so far (42% of vaccinees responding) with the higher DNA dose (5 mg) at the 30-week timepoint. The adenovirus-based candidate shows much stronger immunogenicity and about 67% of the volunteers responding overall, depending on the vaccine dose and the individual's level of pre-existing immunity to adenovirus, a common virus that in its natural form causes colds. These T cell responses appear to recognize antigens including those present in the vaccine, subtype B, and also from several different HIV subtypes. Future studies will focus on:

• Attempting to overcome pre-existing immunity to adenovirus by careful dosing and possibly by using a prime-boost strategy of a DNA prime and adenovirus boost.

(The adenovirus is not in its "natural form" in the vaccines and the genetically engineered adenovirus is an unnatural virulent adenovirus that can cause tumors, and in the study the adenovirus infected 67% of the volunteers guised as "immunogenicity". The Future studies will focus on "attempting to overcome pre-existing immunity to adenovirus", thereby saying future studies will battle the immune system and "overcome pre-existing immunity" to a disease causing pathogen and thereby infect greater than 67% of the volunteers. The vaccines in current studies are intended to "overcome" the natural immune system's responses to the vaccine viruses, that result in infections.)

A Report
www.nih.gov

Says;

Since retroviruses can remain latent in the host by nature of their replication cycle the introduction of a known or unknown retrovirus into humans means that infection if transmitted will become endemic in humans.

The Oxford University Press dictionary definition of endemic: (of a disease or condition) regularly found among particular people or in a certain area.

(Not only is the current use of genetic engineering being misused with antigen and species based devastation and the splicing, sequencing and integration of species cells into live humans is a reality that is notably being left unnoticed by an uninformed public. This misuse of genetic engineering is being left unchecked to grow wild in devastation and the Bush Administration's agendas of isolation and separation of individuals and communities will be escalated with compartmentalizing cross species of humans and animals while at the same time increasing the Bush Administration, as well as existing and following predecessors's influence and power.

The Report titled Plenery Discussion - Future Directions located at www.nih.gov Says;

Some mice contract certain viral infections that cause predictable death in a laboratory setting, however the same viral infection may run a different course in nature.

Acquisition of human hosts by a virus requires an environment conducive for infections, transmission , and establishment of the zoonotic infection of the host.

A Report
Determination of a Statistically Valid Neutralization Titer in Plasma That Confers Protection Against Simian-Human Immunodeficiency Virus Challenge Following Passive Transfer of High-Titered Neutralizing Antibodies www.vrc.nih.gov Says;

There is abundant evidence that a robust antiviral cellular responses are elicited following human immunodeficiency virus type 1 (HIV-1) and simian immunodeficiency virus (SIV) infections of humans and macaques, respectively. This is the pattern observed for most retro-virus infections, which typically become chronic and, in the case of the primate lentiviruses, result in debilitating and fatal clinical outcomes.

A Report Titled; A Partnership for Health: Minorities and Biomedical Research located at www.niaid.nih.gov/publications/minorityhealth.pdf says under the heading Microbiology and Infectious Diseases

Says;

Data from animal model studies includes a greater diversity of vaccine approaches being tested and more products in the pipeline than ever before including a large number of non-clade B products. Specifically the NIH Dale and Betty Bumpers VRC and NIAID's HIV Vaccine Design and Development Teams are moving strong HIV vaccine candidates from the laboratory into human testing.

A report titled Dateline NIAID, June 1996 Disarmed HIV Delivers Genes to Rat Neurons
www.niaid.nih.gov/publications/dateline/full/0696.htm

Says;

Vectors made from modified, nonpathogenic viruses are essential tools in gene therapy. Scientists splice corrective genes into vectors and then infect diseased or damaged cells with the custom-made constructs.

The Report titled "Factors Which Restrict Post-Entry Stages of Pathogenesis" www.nih.gov
http://www.nih.gov

Says;

The ability of viral gene products to interact with human proteins could thus represent "predictors of transmissibility."

(The viral gene products are the "predictors of transmissibility" and not sex being the predominate "predictor of transmissibility" as exploited and advertised. The continued development of repetitive genetically engineered SHIV chimeric viruses to be distributed to infect innocent individuals is because of the big business of HIV/AIDS and "me too" vaccine corporations and associated players of the HIV/AIDS charade wanting a piece of the pie in the HIV/AIDS big picture agenda.)

The International AIDS Vaccine Initiative glossary definition of genetic engineering and recombinant located on pages 46 and 48 of the 2002 Annual Progress Report at www.iavi.org/viewpage.cfm?aid=34 is

Genetic Engineering: The laboratory technique of splicing together genes to produce specific proteins, for example to use as vaccines or medicines.

Recombinant: A cell or an individual with a new combination of genes not found together in either parents; usually applied to linked genes. See genetic engineering

The NIAID Vaccine glossary definition of Recombinant DNA Technology located at http://www.niaid.nih.gov/factsheets/glossary.htm

recombinant DNA technology: the technique by which genetic material from one organism is inserted into a foreign cell in order to mass produce the protein encoded by the inserted genes.

A Report Under Vaccines titled Recombinant Vaccinia Virus Vaccines dated 6/9/2004 located at
http.www.ncbi.nlm.nih.gov/books/bv.fcgi?rid=vacc.section.53 or www.ncbi.nlm.nih.gov

Says;

Recombinant vaccinia viruses provide a powerful means of dissecting the immune responses of humans and experimental animals to individual gene products of infectious agents.

A clinical trial
Safety of Recombinant HIV Vaccines in HIV Infected Young Adults on Stable Therapy
http://www.clinicaltrials.gov/ct/show/NCT00107549?order=4

Says;

The purpose of this study is to determine the safety of 4 recombinant HIV vaccines in HIV infected young adults on stable anti-HIV therapy.

In HIV infected young adults who have well controlled HIV replication on highly active antiretroviral therapy (HAART), the two pairs of matching recombinant HIV-1 vaccines that utilize a modified vaccinia Ankara (MVA) vector and a fowlpox vector (FPV) will be used. Development of any adverse events of Grade 3 or higher; development of adverse events of Grade 3 or higher attributed to the study vaccines; viral breakthrough to greater than 1,000 copies/ml within the first 26 weeks on study. Exclusion Criteria: Prior vaccination with any HIV-1 vaccine

Prior vaccination against smallpox

Prior vaccinia immunization

In addition, Males enrolled in the study must use a condom from the first vaccination until one month after the last vaccination.

A Study

SHIV transmission and susceptibility to re-exposure through social contact Following vaccination with an HIV synthetic peptide-cocktail www.blackwell-synergy.com

Says;

Although an earlier study of rhesus macaques indicated that SIV could not be detected in cultures of semen samples, a more recent study of pig-tailed macaques verified the expression of SHIV in the semen during primary infection.

(The above clinical trial using genetically engineered (recombinant) vaccinia HIV and instructing the Males enrolled in the study to use a condom from the first vaccination until one month after the last vaccination is once again, the government and the pharmaceutical industry intentionally infecting individuals in clinical trials. Some genetically engineered viruses are only "verified" during "primary infection and as a result in the above study the objective was direct infection of the targeted individuals only in the clinical trial and not an objective of generating transmissibility of the genetically engineered viruses via sexual intercourse ever.

Currently sex is not the primary mode of transmissibility of HIV/SIV (SHIV) even during the primary infection period, but the longer they are allowed to experiment on humans and animals the greater the likelihood sex could become a form of transmissibility targeting for example, Gay couples unable to marry, and vulnerable to more harassing stigma and societal complacency of the government and co-sponsored deadly disease causing antigens causing more discrimination and hate crimes along the way on a long and arduous mis-guided direction of power over the masses ultimately embedding more formalized Globalization juncture and disparity in slavery.)

A Report
Factors Affecting Infectious Agent Pathogenicity
www.nih.gov
Says;

Explore innovative trial designs to improve efficiency of vaccine efficacy studies. Determine the impact of HIV vaccines on subsequent transmission from vaccinated individuals who become infected after administration of the trial vaccine utilizing initially concordant negative couples at "high risk" or discordant couples.

The Jordan Report
www.niaid.nih.gov/dmid/vaccines/jordan20/jordan20_2002.pdf

Says;

The greatest public health value of a vaccine will be its ability to prevent transmission.

The National Institutes of Health Fiscal Year 2003 Plan For HIV Related Research www.oar.nih.gov/public/pubs/fy2003/iii_etiology.pdf

Says;

Emphasis should be placed on studies focused on groups of people that are most representative of the expanding HIV epidemic. This can be facilitated by studies whose design reflects the collaboration of basic scientists and population based researchers. There also should be an emphasis on enabling the availability of emerging technologies in genetics, functional genomics and proteomics, and the assessment of host responses for studies of the biology of HIV transmission.

A report
National Institute for Health Fiscal Year 2001 Plan for HIV-Related
Research" located at www.nih.gov/od/oar/public/pubs/fy2001pln.pdf

Says;

Defining the impact of different vaccine approaches on immune
responses and localization of viral replication, long-term followup of
disease progression with low-level chronic infection and biological
characteristics of breakthrough virus including transmissibility.

A Report
Poxvirus-based vaccine candidates for HIV:
Two Decades of experience with special emphasis on canarypox
vectors. www.ncbi.nih.gov

Says;

Poxvirus vectors have emerged as important vectors for licensed
veterinary vaccines and candidate vaccines for humans. Vaccinia, highly attenuated vaccinia strains and avipoxviruses have been assessed extensively in preclinical models, as well as in humans, to determine their
immunogenicity and protective efficacy against HIV. The attenuated
vaccinia strains and avipoxviruses have been shown to be able to carry
HIV genes and express their proteins to induce both antibodies and
cellular immune responses.

The NIH National Center for Research Resources
www.ncrr.nih.gov/newspub/apr02rpt/stories6.asp
Stories of Discovery
Monkey Viruses and Human AIDS

Says;

More than 20 years ago—as concerns about a mysterious and deadly
new disease known as acquired immunodeficiency syndrome (AIDS)
began to sweep the nation—scientists at the California Regional Pri-

mate Research Center (RPRC) were puzzling over an outbreak of infections that were decimating their monkey colonies. Inexplicably, dozens of animals became dangerously thin and weak, and many developed malignant tumors, severe herpesvirus or bacterial infections, anemia, or inflammation of brain tissues. Most affected animals were dead in a matter of months. Meanwhile, on the other side of the country, researchers at the New England RPRC near Boston noticed a similarly disturbing trend among their macaque monkeys.

The Report titled
"The current Status of HIV-1 Vaccine Development, 2004: Recomendations for the Future by The NIAID AIDS Vaccine Research Working Group"
www.niaid.nih.gov/daids/vaccine/pdf/AVRWG/finalreport.pdf

Says;

Genetic variation of HIV-1 is a major obstacle for AIDS vaccine development. Since HIV-1 group M began its expansion in humans approximately 70 years ago, it has diversified rapidly, and now comprises a number of different subtypes and circulating recombinant forms.

Again at the report titled;
Panel Session I: Cross-Species Transmission – Species Specificity and Tropism http://www.niaid.nih.gov/dait/cross-species/page3.htm

Says;

A porcine cell expresses a retrovirus, it infects a human cell . . . and produces a virus capable of transmission to the general public. Complex recombinations do occur, but they are not common.

A Report located Under Vaccines at Recombinant Vaccinia Virus Vaccines dated 6/9/2004 http.www.ncbi.nlm.nih.gov/books/bv.fcgi?rid=vacc.section.53 or www.ncbi.nlm.nih.gov

Says;

Procedures developed for the construction of recombinant vaccinia viruses have been applied to members of other poxvirus genera including avian poxviruses and capripoxviruses. Eventhough the avian poxviruses are naturally host range restricted, gene expression and protective immunity can be established in nonavian species.

(Not only are viruses being intentionally introduced into targeted individuals and communities, but the resulting diseases are labeled HIV/AIDS, and the pending so-called Avian Flu Virus pandemic is being created in the same manner to unnaturally introduce infectious agents into the human population, but unlike HIV/AIDS patients not labeled HIV have a better chance of survival in the "real world." The "avian poxviruses are naturally host range restricted", and the original SIV virus which is a simian virus that was host range restricted and caused no disease until man genetically engineered the virus and transplanted the altered virus into both simians and humans to cross infect and mutate a virus to manifest into AIDS to perpetuate the current ongoing deadly mood of protective lies hidden in deadly vaccines and medicines. The phrase "gene expression and protective immunity can be established in nonavian species" when there is no natural reason to establish so-called "protective immunity" of "host range restricted" viruses is the same pretense as the HIV virus was altered to infect across species and expressed the altered gene into humans. The American laboratory warfare is creating all types of pathogenic viruses (many of which are labeled HIV) designed to attack certain individuals and communities to be unwanted hosts in the American community of Stepford people up with the Jonses of flagrance and arrogance to unwittingly perpetuate sick and tired all around the world.)

A Report
Panel Session II: Cross-Species Transmission Mechanisms of Pathogen Adaptation www.vrc.nih.gov/dait/cross-species/pages6.htm

Says;

Avian influenza viruses are perpetuated in aquatic birds and oc-
casionally transmit to other host species. Periodically they transmit to
humans indirectly through pigs.

The Report titled;
Panel Session I: Cross-Species Transmission – Species Specificity
and Tropism
www.nih.gov

Says;

Researchers are beginning to assess pig viruses for pig into human
viral transmission.

It is possible that genetically modified pigs would be more capable
of cross-species viral transmission and aborgation of hyperacute rejection will make pig envelope viruses more resistant to inactivation by
human complement with some viruses being possibly pre-adapted for
transfer to humans.

The Report titled
Resources for HIV Vaccine Research and Development
www.thebody.com/niaid/resources.html
Genetic Sequence Variability of HIV-1 and Related Lentiviruses
Says; The contract currently held by the University of Alabama at Bir-
mingham carries out genetic cloning and sequencing studies. Through
the contract full length proviruses representing clades A through H
(group M subtypes), a number of subtype recombinant viruses and several group O viruses have been cloned and sequenced in their entirety.
Individual viral genes have been subcloned into expresion vectors as
research tools. These clones can be used to produce proteins in various expression systems for the creation of SIV-HIV chimeric viruses
(SHIV) or directly in design of vaccines. In addition, gag, pol, env, and
nef genes from clades A through H have been subcloned into shuttle
vectors for generating recombinant vaccinia viruses.

A Report
Challenges in Designing HIV Vaccines
www.niaid.nih.gov/factsheets/challvacc.htm

Says;

Genes encoding the envelope and core proteins of HIV isolates obtained from patients have been analyzed and compared. Scientists have grouped HIV isolates obtained from patients have also been analyzed and compared. And as a result, scientists have grouped HIV isolates worldwide into three groups, M, N. And O. The M (Major) group can be further divided into 9 subtypes. Each subtype within a group is about 30 percent different from any of the others. If an individual is infected with two different subtypes a new (recombinant) form of virus can result that contains gene fragments from both parental viruses. Hence there are an infinite number of HIV variants circulating worldwide, and a successful vaccine will need to induce an immune response that protects against a large portion of these variants.

A Report
The current Status of HIV-1 Vaccine Development, 2004:
Recomendations for the Future by The NIAID AIDS Vaccine Research Working Group
www.niaid.nih.gov/daids/vaccine/pdf/AVRWG/finalreport.pdf

Says;

Recombination occurs frequently, and a circulating recombinant form (CRF) carries sections of two or more
HIV-1 subtypes in a mosaic genome.

(If someone is infected with two different subtypes or strains a new (recombinant) form of virus can result that contains gene fragments from both parental viruses with an infinite number of HIV variants circulating worldwide is what is occurring in the intentional vaccine and medicine induced infections worldwide creating a monster that has to be fed. In addition, the Bush Administration along with the so-called "AIDS Vaccine Enterprise" are trying to create an infrastructure of many vaccines being used throughout the world to ultimately infiltrate   regions, separate via disease segregation and gain control by emerging diseases of containment. The fact that the first vaccine trial in Africa in 1999 was not based on an HIV clade prevalent in Africa and then just 2 years later the researchers and scientists invaded Africa again with vaccines and personnel that were "re-tooled" as human delivery weapons based on a new agenda of HIV clade prevalent agendas of intense segregation and no scrutiny in Africa or anywhere around the world. The more confusion to create geographical diversity of viruses connected to humans the more humans will not care about other humans. "Esparza recognized, however, that there is some uncertainty regarding the relevance of HIV subtypes in AIDS vaccine induced protection" is because the only relevance is adding additional genetically engineered recombinations to the vaccines filled to "include the sequences of breakthrough isolates from all HIV-1 vaccine trials" to propagate more variants of the so-called HIV virus and stigmatize more communities in the never ending and ever growing HIV/AIDS charade.)

The Clinical Trial titled; "Safety of and Immune Response to Polyvalent HIV-1 Vaccine in HIV Uninfected Adults"
  http://clinicaltrials.gov/ct/show/NCT00061243?order=3

Says;

Two HIV antigens, Gag and Env, are included in this study's vaccine formulation. Studies have shown that HIV-1 Gag is a potent inducer of cell mediated immune responses, while ENV is the target of neutralizing antibody responses. The vaccine used in this study contains a 5-valent ENV design (ENV derived from one of 5 clades of HIV) in order to examine if a polyvalent Env formulation may expand the breadth of neutralizing antibody responses induced in human volunteers.

For both DNA priming and protein boosting, a set of Env antigens from clades A,B,C, and E of HIV-1 M group will be produced (2Env antigens from clade B and 1 Env each from the other three clades). All 5 Env antigens are selected from the primary HIV-1 viral isolates with the hope of producing broad antibody responses against the primary viruses circulating in the worldwide human population.

A Report
Human Immunodeficiency Virus-1 Envelope Glycoproteins and Anti-CD4 Antibodies Inhibit Interleukin-2-Induced Jak/STAT signalling in Human CD4 T Lymphocytes
www.blackwell-synergy.com

Says;

The recombinant HIV-1 envelope glycoprotein (env) used in all experiments was obtained from Pasteur-Merieux Connaught (Marcy l'Etoile, France) in purified form. The gp120 and gp41 portions of the preparation were derived from MN and LAI strains of HIV-1. At the concentrations used, env proteins were able to saturate CD4 on the cell surface as determined by the elimination of anti-CD4-FITC antibodies (MT310, Dako, Glostrup, Denmark) binding by flow cytometry.

(The elimination of anti-CD4-FITC antibodies along with the statement above in the hope of producing broad antibody responses against the primary viruses circulating in the worldwide human population is the facade of the HIV/AIDS Vaccine Enterprise charade and the lies involved in inducing false hope with antibodies that are abused with the working part of the vaccines being virus and bacteria recombinations labeled HIV. In addition, creating new recombinations such as the above using the gp120 and gp41 portions of the preparation derived from MN and LAI strains of HIV-1.)

The definition of gp41 located at The NAID HIV Vaccine Glossary http://www.niaid.nih.gov/factsheets/glossary.htm

gp41: glycoprotein 41. A protein imbedded in the outer envelope of HIV that anchors gp120. gp41 plays a key role in HIV's infection of

CD4 T cells by facilitating the fusion of the viral and cell membranes. Antibodies to gp41 can be detected on a screening HIV Elisa.

MN: an HIV-1 strain belonging to clade B, the clade to which most HIV-1 found in North America and Europe belong. MN is used in vaccine development."(See also clade.)

Isolate: a particular strain of HIV-1 taken from a person.

strain: one type of HIV. HIV is so heterogeneous, no two isolates are exactly the same. When HIV is isolated from an individual, and worked on in the lab, it is given its own unique identifier or strain name (i.e. MN, LAI).

LAI: an HIV isolate used in HIV vaccine development. LAI is also referred to as IIIB or LAV. LAI belongs to clade B, the clade to which most HIV-1 found in america and Europe belongs.

subtype: also called a clade. With respect to HIV isolates, a classification scheme based on genetic differences.

polyvalent vaccine: a vaccine that is produced from multiple viral strains, or is made to induce immune responses against multiple strains.

The International Aids Vaccine Initiative website located at www.iavi.org under the side heading of "IAVI Database of AIDS Vaccines in Human Trial" then search for all vaccines ever tested and the company

GlaxoSmithKline vaccine is a combination of recombinant proteins formed into an adjuvanted multi-antigen vaccine.

The Report titled;
"National Institute for Health Fiscal Year 2001 Plan for HIV-Related Research" located at www.nih.gov/od/oar/public/pubs/fy2001pln.pdf

Says;

Multivalent vaccine candidates incorporating different genetic clades and antigentic types to increase breadth of immune responses.

A Workshop Report
Rhesus Monkey Demands
in Biomedical Researchwww.ncrr.nih.gov/compmed/rhesuswork-shopreport.pdf

Says;

The most consistent AIDS model in the pigtail non-human primate is infection with HIV-2287. This model always leads to AIDS and has a realistic time frame and is good for testing antiviral drugs. Pigtails are remarkably susceptible to SHIVs and can even be infected with HIV-1 but the persistence of infection and the level of viral load are not sufficient to evaluate vaccines.

The Report of
The current Status of HIV-1 Vaccine Development, 2004: Recomendations for the Future by The NIAID AIDS Vaccine Research Working Group"
    www.niaid.nih.gov/daids/vaccine/pdf/AVRWG/finalreport.pdf

Says;

Define protection to HIV in other animal models of SIV/SHIV infection and in human clinical trials.

A Workshop Report
Rhesus Monkey Demands
in Biomedical Research
www.ncrr.nih.gov/compmed/rhesusworkshopreport.pdf

Says;

More lentivirus challenge studies should be conducted using alternative macaque models, including Chinese rhesus, cynomolgus, and pigtailed macaques. And more challenge studies should be conducted with SHIV because the number of HIV recombinants is growing and researchers cannot predict either their behavior or their virulence.

National Institutes of Health Fiscal Year 2001 Plan for HIV-Related Research PREPARED BY THE DIRECTOR OFFICE OF AIDS RESEARCH NATIONAL INSTITUTES OF HEALTH www.nih.gov/od/oar/public/pubs/fy2001pln.pdf

Says;

Rhesus macaques have presented particular opportunities for assessment of HIV/simian immunodeficiency virus (SIV) vaccine strategies because of the development of disease from SIV in this model and the adaptation of several pathogenic SHIV chimeric isolates. Generation of additional SHIV chimeric isolates for vaccine applications allows the direct evaluation of vaccine candidates with HIV envelope components for different types or clades of HIV-1 isolates.

The Report titled;
National Institute for Health Fiscal Year 2001 Plan for HIV-Related Research located at www.nih.gov/od/oar/public/pubs/fy2001pln

Says;

There is a selection of viral antigens for the design of an HIV vaccine and using viral and microbial antigens in animal and humans are being used to develop optimal vaccine strategies for HIV antigen delivery.

(HIV/AIDS is not a result of so-called HIV but rather various viruses being genetically engineered using different hosts to harvest and concoct more varying mutated antigens to deliver into more targeted individuals and communities being chastised, advertised, labeled and judged as societal poison.)

A Report titled;
"National Institute for Health Fiscal Year 2001 Plan for HIV-Related Research" located at www.nih.gov/od/oar/public/pubs/fy2001pln.pdf

Design and conduct Phase I and Phase II trials using promising HIV vaccine candidates that are genetically or immunologically related to HIV isolates circulating in a proposed trial population. Trials should address questions that test vaccine concepts, include an appropriate representation of ethnic and racial minority populations affected by HIV, and be of an appropriate size to provide data on the frequency of immune responses to facilitate decisions regarding initiation and evaluation of larger "proof of concept" or efficacy trials.

(The American government is intentionally developing organisms in individuals to be classified and set apart by disease. The AIDS epidemic amongst homosexual men being categorized by government hating and spreading disease is a disgusting behavior.)

A Report titled
The current Status of HIV-1 Vaccine Development, 2004: Recommendations for the Future by The NIAID AIDS Vaccine Research Working Group
www.niaid.nih.gov/daids/vaccine/pdf/AVRWG/finalreport.pdf

Says;

Build community information and education dissemination in the plans for continued trial network development to ensure that expectations of the community are realistic.

A variety of community preparedness approaches and materials were presented. Several posters documented the connection between community education and engagement with AIDS vaccine trial recruitment.

A Report
Changing American's Attitudes Towards HIV Vaccine Research
A Community-Based Approach
Division of AIDS/NIAID/NIH, Bethesda, MD, United States
Says;

Given that a phase III efficacy trial will require tens of thousands of volunteers efforts such as this campaign will need to be continued along with similar programs likely to be beneficial in other locales.

A Report
The National Academies Press NAP's Skim View of: The Genomic Revolution: Eugenics, the Genome, and Human Rights
http://www.nap.edu

Says;

Explore the ramifications of the Human Genome Project and address the social, economic, and ethical impacts of advancing genetic technologies and their effect on our understanding of natural history.

In the United States it fostered so-called Fitter Family competitions, a standard feature at several state fairs that were held in their human stock sections. At the 1924 Kansas Free Fair winning families in the three categories small, average, and large were awarded a Governor's Fitter Family Trophy. In Alabama, for example, attempts to pass a sterilization law in the mid-1930s prompted a Methodist newspaper to warn that the proposed sterilization bill is steep toward the totalitarianism in Germany today. The state is taking private matters of individual conscience, and matters of family control in hand, and sometimes it's a rough hand, and always it's a strong hand.

(The Bush Administration and their Neo-Nazi conservative ideals of hate and abuse are currently abusing the Genome Project in attempts to foster so-called winning families and human stocks of the future by amplifying a thousand fold of the already destructive nature in bigotry and discrimination in lab science that creates Firm Hand HIV viruses today that are far from a human hand trying to shake off the feelings

inside of betrayal and loss of life. That type of direction and manipulation will only create a laughing stock of the human race and end any
laughter that is from the heart while fostering only nervous tension
to laugh. Laughing at mother nature is not funny and any winning
families created by the Genome Project will be inappropriately judged
by the heart as losers that create altruistic wars. HIV/AIDS making a
difference in a lifestyle to live differently under a Bush Administration
military environment controlling people is genetic tragedy engineering to rape life on the sly out of spite to be internalized all the while
Bush wacked unable to be a fit family altogether to grow into the fabric
of life. The Bush Administration and co-sponsors of "fitter families"
decimating animals and humans to advertise a superiority complex are
intense hate crimes of scale out of balance of Gays unable to adopt unwanted children as not a fit family unwanted is the inner child in all of
us wanting life to be more than less friendly by the misuse of genetics
advocating "fitter families" concept of the early 1920's decimating life
to come and go freedom never in step with time.

Genetics today with a future of "fitter families" pronounced twisting down the road for a mutated tomorrow is an infrastructure of isolation and laws of discrimination and segregation building today by
arrogance setting the stage for more down the road more loss and more
heartache. The current Bush Administration years having the most
HIV/AIDS "related" deaths year after year in fit "minority" communities trying to walk out of Silence = Death is a gap between spirituality
and evil health care. Where is the true future for true happiness to
move a sense of well being forward as a new age of grounded happiness
and peace to be a resource today and tomorrow to see the road as joy
instead of the road before us as more underground pain to be unfurled
to maneuver around going where? Isolation, discrimination and segregation as an infrastructure today to be cattle prodded down the road
for the right winged hate monger's tomorrow is excruciating pain and
slavery needing abolishment today for freedom to heal our wounds.
Silence = Death is a no freedom war zone sign of the times today dismal living. Interactions with good friends are necessary for friends to
live and learn in freedom as a gift of life to be electric and spontaneous

without the control of laboratory HIV/AIDS strategies in the millions decimating the atmosphere.

Life should not be so arduously unequal living lopsided and if education and freedom could connect to give structure to Christmas as a family tree our heritage would have more meaning each day as a new day of spiritual expectations of growth that are not daunting on Christmas one day. Faith awareness dates back to Jesus, Mary Magdalen and Gay Indians spanning the gamut of spiritual love as a cultural norm easily to understand love and forgiveness in spiritual grounding not a religion of petty grievances never instilling into society a true spirit of life. Sport teams with Indian names without the dignity of an Indian prayer is insane not to recognize true ancestry on and off the field of respect for the human race. Tribal or music are not the same today a gap of song and a prayer to be rhythmic in spirit forgotten the beat is in the heart not the thunder of attitudes of winning at all costs for "fitter families" on the sport field flood war chants after a National Anthem.

An Indian prayer includes nature and spirit yet the American National Anthem includes bombs and the twilights last gleaming. Sad is the American song in thin air on thin ice shooting off rockets melting remnants of stability being replaced with a safety of conservative compassionate conservancy culture awareness today is all consuming not faith awareness of being one with nature and spirituality singing and chanting all inclusive in a field of view of spirituality is no accident in nature. Worlds apart from the Bush Administration is pure joy in a real moment like this few and far between the constant harassing attrition strategies of no real relief unless meditating to stop and smell the roses in conjunction with trying to expose the truth of the HIV/AIDS charade where senses are heightened to chant no more years of repressiveness living around the Bush Administration trying to create a culture for their safety while decimating our safety of real concerns.

A multitude of problems caused by the HIV/AIDS charade and the Bush Administration wants to "more frequently" include the Gay community to more frequently attend our own funeral processions is a long road with many problems and relief is difficult in environmental control to the grave. Where is the relief? We need to end the constant unnecessary problems that batters our bodies, minds and souls today in a procession of dead bodies from laboratory diseases and evil harassing strategies that wastes so much valuable time living in space of Silence = Death.)

A report titled Mouse Model Mimics Real-World Plague Infection located at

http://www.niaid.nih.gov/Newsroom/Releases/plaguemouse.htm

says;

Replicating the natural transmission of plague from flea to host in this model is tedious and unusual work notes NIAID Director Anthony S. Fauci, M.D. This approach, however, brings researchers much closer to answers to real-life questions. It is difficult to do a natural challenge for an arthropod-transmitted disease. You have to have flea colonies. You have to be able to infect them safely. You need medical entomology, microbiology and biosafety expertise. It is much easier to infect a host artificially with a needle and syringe. Plague has been used as a bioweapon before and it could be again.

A Workshop Report
"Rhesus Monkey Demands
in Biomedical Research"
www.ncrr.nih.gov/compmed/rhesusworkshopreport.pdf

Says;

A survey of studies published from 1999 to 2002 of live lentivirus SIV, SHIV, HIV-1, HIV-2 challenges to vaccinated nonhuman primates indicates that most of the challenges are being done intravenously,

A Report titled Plenery Discussion Future Directions
located at www.nih.gov
Says;

The most serious, albeit less likely, event is the potential to generate a new epidemic by introducing nonhuman infectious agents into the human population.

Again the Report titled;
The Genomic Revolution: Unveiling The Unity of Life
http://books.nap.edu/books/0309074363/html/196.html

Says;

Genetic information can be used to classify and lump, split and separate, identify and admit. Many nations have , for example, granted the right of return if you can show that your ancestors come from a particular place. Citizenship often keys on biological inheritance. In the future genetics will interest those social, scientific, anthropological, and even archeological areas in very interesting ways.

(Did Jesus an ancester come from a particular place or was Jesus murdered in a particular place to be granted a right to return policy? The biological inheritance has always been now but soon planned by expensive agendas mutated in hyper-space of the now biological inheritance will rapidly mutate and evolve biological inheritance to be based on manipulated genetics and discrimination. The Judas segment of conservancy wants to replace natural with confusion and convolution of evolution trying ignorantly to replace Jesus with murder today as a figment for riches gone wild tomorrow for a few that will not be buried on earth of real riches as long as as the conservancy is searching for their riches not to love. Trust and faith is far removed from the "evangelical" labeled as intense Christianity separated by Catholic Christianity all the same in riches amputated for a label of lost love that only names separate themselves as a concept of love lost in Jesus on earth today giving only to the people that cry to be save from Judas regardless of money. When will we learn that the credit of Jesus spreading love is smothered in layers that the stone hearts of "Christian Easter Day" are not willing to roll away the stone in process of manipulation biologically evolving Judas "biologically" polluting the spirit to levitate insensitivities of the rich leveraging to roll away the stone of captivity to give not the poor to be abused without any resources and tricked to give the shirt off our backs, but to give to Jesus and God unconditionally to learn from our giving that Jesus and God already have? What purpose does a mutant mouse or a knock-out pig serve but to label rich biologically possessed? How many monkeys in researched cages above and beyond the monkeys wired shut in more questions than evidence could ever cover-up are needed before we are knocked out un-conscience in a quagmire of swallowing the lies along with the dissatisfaction? Did Jesus live in biology? Was Jesus rich with biology or was Jesus God before extinction? Distinguishing the "conservancy" movement is simple with love of our sense of trust in God and Jesus not loving ignorance of the "conservancy" agendas cracking down on peanuts for their own elephant nature that is designed to control the love of real elephants in nature wanting only abundance in food to grow in love of difference as a long time Jesus is wanting to join us with His father before death. Safe and Sound and not to biologically "sound off" in praises of "conservancy" elephants sounding politically inept not remembering whole heartedly of what Jesus gave to denounce Judas to wipe away all tears still today dying for simple survival full of resources walled off by the ignorant mis-use of trust. The problem of the 9/11 G. Bush strategy along with the growing agenda of the HIV/AIDS charade is more wedges to chew carve out trust and force denouncement of trust setting us back brain washed and brain dead not to remember Jesus, but to contemplate a flag burning or snow mobiles in National Parks or Gays being ambushed together on a snow mobile in a National park of crimes extending into a biological park.

Biological riches of peanut brain dreams is more captivity and manipulation of nature within an infrastructure being built as a world class zoo around nature. Real elephants and donkeys of importance as people wanting freedom the same opposed frustrated by the importance of ignorant wealth in captivity is a world in captivity. Around and around the politicians are caging their own in servitude unaware of the boxed corner building for centuries one box inside of another to look down at captivity bigger smaller with more or less freedom granted than the stupid corner office unaware that the fire within misdirected to build better boxes angers to shake the visualized people below in condescending order to waste everyone's time.

To be free outside of boxes towering in all directions without having to think how to stay outside of the box and still stay alive is unnatural. Unfortunately, in America our days being numbered are greater today under the rule of the Bush Administration and company detailing and refining boxes never allowed to think for self preservation as a healthy thinking person on all twos standing slumped over is all too familiar in abusing science to abuse man to be sick and depressed. The elephant in the board room mentality is complete and total disaster of a person that is sad messy but builds the best boxes. Where is the love? Where is the freedom to carve out a tiny space of unobstructed views of no business to satisfy only love boxed in or not as long as there is real love to flourish without obstruction of privacy? Forced to make choices to satisfy others as a way of self preservation is self mutilation not to be happy and someday rise by no other choice of aspiration in a subset of destroyed dreams within a no-fault society to be sacrificial lambs and corporate citizens laying down agreements to self to be a simpletons in niche cubicles cornered bored to tears alone bleeding for time to be giving self better un-compromised. The elephant in the room signifying abuse is only in a bigger cage side by side the subordinate monkeys that already realize longevity was long gone on all levels yesterday. A shelter is many boxes already built, but to find shelter in compromise is a lonely box still built by society to compromise immunity. To shelter oneself because of dreams that are suppose to be contained, but trying nonetheless, is foul play falling from above forced by the handy work of government and industry boxes built from the ground up that demand our attention not to waver, but stand still and mutate speech and expression to put a noose around our necks or a drop of a mouse trap over our heads to become docile domesticated subservient human multitudes. What are we suppose to do with our energy? I am so tired of running to be free. Why can we not build a habitat for humanity instead of more shelters? Wetlands set aside as bird sanctuaries or a place for animals for refuge is a habitat, so why we do have to feel being isolated as fish in a barrel building our habitat waiting to be shot? Are we that ashamed of ourselves as a whole? Thousands of new mouse species existing because of mad science and because "genetic information can be used to classify and lump, split and separate, identify and admit"to be on the dismal horizon of the future to be second generational of more preverse discrimination and segregation in humans once the transfer of "genes and proteins found across animal species" have been integrated into the DNA of a significant number of humans and the mutated human models evolve to be even more controlled than enclosure in a cubicle is morbidity. Animals of all species will enabled cross-species disease to humans and on and on the mutants will slowly become us.)

The Mission Statements under
The Nature Conservancy's Values
www.nature.org/aboutus/features

Says;

It is indispensable to The Nature Conservancy's success as our unifying mission, vision, goals and measures as unique values and distinguishing attributes that characterize how we conduct ourselves in a drive for tangible, lasting results. The Nature's Conservancy is aware of the needs of local communities by developing ways to conserve biological diversity while at the same time enabling humans to live productively and sustainably on the landscape. We know that lasting conservation success requires the active involvement of individuals from diverse backgrounds and beliefs and the unique contributions that each person can make to the Nature's Conservancy's cause.

AIDS Vaccines for the World: Working Together to Accelerate Development and Delivery www.iavi.org/file.cfm?fid=394

Says;

Social science research and outreach to communities should underlie the process creating the opportunity to change the trend of scientific research so that communities and ultimately all of us can benefit.

(The Bush Administration and company are launching a global vaccine initiative as directed by the administration with stepped-up resources and destructive obscurities so the unique contributions that each person can make to a cause is in alignment to literally lay down and die for government and industry so ultimately all of them can benefit to control the world.)

2004 G8 Summit report located at-
http://www.whitehouse.gov/news/releases/2004/06/20040610-5.html

Says;

Barry Bennett extolled all of us to say thank you to the volunteers. Lots of these local citizens and others have come here to make your lives easier and to serve you food and drive you around and give you access and help serve you. And would just ask that we follow today if you see these local folks just say "thank you" because they really have done a great job for you and for the summit and for these leaders -- a lot of long hours. They are all volunteers and they do not get paid. As a matter of fact, it is costing them more than they would ever get out of it. So just thank them today if you see them because they want to help you.

As a next step is what can we do about the development of a vaccine which is a very problematic issue because of the scientific gaps, as well as the logistic gaps. A group of scientists, in the summer of '03, put together a broad proposal in a paper that was published in Science Magazine in June of 2003, calling for the need for a global HIV enterprise, which a virtual consortium and not an organization with a head and with pooled money, but an agreement to form an alliance among the interested stakeholders, be they individual scientists, government or what have you, to agree upon the philosophy that we will develop a strategic plan that would provide coordination, collaboration, and sharing of information, as well as closing the gaps.

The President proposed this to the G8, and the G8 has endorsed this global HIV enterprise, which to emphasize a virtual consortium based on a strategic plan so that when other nations, G8 and other nations, decide they want to align their own resources or put new resources into vaccine development, there will be a strategic plan framework with which they can synergize with the other nations.

Each individual country will own their own resources. This is not pooling of resources. It is getting individual entities to agree upon the commitment that they will work in a collaborative way towards an HIV vaccine.

Immediately upon deciding upon that and announcing it G. Bush Jr. wanted to go even further in developing a more global treatment and care program which over the next several months working intensively with White House staff they have put together what is now known as the President's emergency plan for AIDS relief. A $15 billion program that over five years is going to treat 2 million people in 14 countries in sub-Saharan Africa and the Caribbean, and prevent 7 million infections and care for 10 million people.

"This proposal has been endorsed, and as the new announcement associated with this, is that to get the ball rolling in these six major components of the strategic plan, the President is proposing spending $15 million in '05 for a virtual center. Now a virtual center is a center where you have the sort of money that glues people together be it in a medical center, or what have you. And then the '06 money that would be the continuation of that will be decided according to the standard of budgetary process to go through each year.

Funding of the initial virtual center will come through the peer review mechanism and has been agreed upon to have the strategic plan individuals as a global array of individuals reporting within the next several months to the United States as the G8 presidency this year, and then each year, starting with the UK next year and beyond, each year, there will be a reporting of the progress of the strategic plan.

Q. Has any other country put up money here at G8?

DR. FAUCI: Not right now, because they were just met with the agreement of this. This was just put upon them, as the sherpas (stakeholders) got together and worked this out. And now the concept of the enterprise has been agreed upon and endorsed by the G8, and we fully expect and hope that there will be interest in joining and embracing this strategic plan, so that if a company or country comes in they could pick any one, two, three or four or whatever of the six major components of the enterprise, and say, we decide that we would like to get involved in contributing to this.

DR. FAUCI: Will be happy to entertain any questions after, about the initiatives that are going to be made public today in the arena of health. The first one, which is really the new, brand-new deliverable is what is being referred to as the global HIV vaccine enterprise.It is an exciting new initiative and rounds out the approach regarding prevention, care, and, in this case now, treatment, and now, finally, with vaccines.

(If a company and/or a country jumps in with the Bush administration's web of hate labeled as an enterprise then they stand to gain financially. It is a game of control and greed where developing countries are vulnerable to be seized by way of money and disease resulting in the demise of their culture by the big business of HIV/AIDS controlling life being nurtured by a Vaccine Enterprise consisting of government and corporate imbeciles The statement "in this case now, treatment, and now, finally, with vaccines" is mis-treatment and torture of a planned 2 million people and 10 million individuals already in the system of being managed and bilked of their resources by government and industry with a master plan that contains everything but health care forcing people to serve as slaves treated to die off the land. The statements they are all volunteers and they do not get paid and as a matter of fact, it is costing them more than they would ever get out of it. And lots of these local citizens and others have come here to make your lives easier -- to serve you food and drive you around and give you access and help serve you are statements of the true reasons for the development of the "Vaccine Enterprise" and Globalization whereby a volunteer is a slave in the eyes of the global enterprise instigators as snubbed nosed elitists intervening with lethal vaccinations of control and no matter if they are serving food or volunteering in a HIV clinical trial the sad fact is that it is costing more in lives lost than anyone could ever get out of living life. Globalization with the aid of disease is a way the enterprise can control countries and populations, as well as re-emerge slavery on a global scale.)

The Report titled "Reagent Resource Support for AIDS Vaccine Development" located at www.niaid.nih.gov/contract/archive/rfp0301.pdf

Says;

To overcome HIV-1 diversity, "centralized" HIV-1 genes in HIV immunogen design have been proposed. These strategies include using consensus, the most frequent base found in a given position, or ancestral or center of the tree sequences, both modeled from phylogenetic trees. Three computer models (consensus, ancestor, and center of the tree (COT) have been proposed to generate centralized HIV-1 genes.

While consensus sequences are arguably the most representative of the most circulating viral populations, ancestral and COT sequences hypothetically may have an advantage of re-creating potent epitopes that have tended to escape over time during chronic infections, but for reasons of viral fitness and transmission, tend to revert to a more ancestral form in a new host. Data presented at the AIDS Vaccine 2003 meeting established the initial proof of concept that centralized consensus HIV-1 genes can be both antigenic and immunogenic for wild-type epitopes.

A web site, obviously without much elaboration, except a computer program that can direct researchers in their quest for species altercation is exemplified by saying the user can reroot, flip branches, change names of species, change or remove branch lengths, and move around to look at various parts of the tree if it is too large to fit on the screen.: RETREE
www.http://evolution.genetics.washington.edu/phylip/doc/retree.html
or www.evolution.genetics.washington.edu

Niles Stanley

Illustrates;

`<phylogenies> <phylogeny> <clade> <clade length="0.87231"><name>Mouse</name></clade> <clade length="0.49807"><name>Bovine</name></clade> <clade length="0.39538"> <clade length="0.25930"><name>Gibbon</name></clade> <clade length="0.10815"> <clade length="0.24166"><name>Orang</name></clade> <clade length="0.04405"> <clade length="0.12322"><name>Gorilla</name></clade> <clade length="0.06026"> <clade length="0.13846"><name>Chimp</name></clade> <clade length="0.0857"><name>Human</name></clade> </clade> </clade> </clade> </clade> </clade> </phylogeny> </phylogenies>`

The National Institute of Health Vaccine Glossary http://www.niaid.nih.gov/factsheets/glossary.htm definition of

clade: also called a subtype. A group of related HIV isolates classified according to their degree of genetic similarity (such as their envelope proteins). There are currently two groups of HIV-1 isolates, M and O. M consists of at least nine clades, A through I. Group O may consist of a similar number of clades.

Merriam Webster's Medical Desk Dictionary Revisied Edition definitions of

phylogeny: the evolutionary history of a kind of organism
:the evolution of a genetically related group of organisms as distinguished from the development of the individual organism.

phylum: a major group of animals or in some classification plants sharing one or more fundamental characteristics that set them apart from all other animals and plants and forming a primary category of the animal or plant kingdom.

A Report titled;
"High Risk Research" http://nihroadmap.nih.gov/highrisk/index.asp

140

Says;

The NIH Roadmap has created a new funding program, the NIH Director's Pioneer Award, to encourage creative, outside-the-box thinkers to pursue exciting and innovative ideas about biomedical research. Awardees will have the intellectual freedom to pursue their ideas and follow them in expected or even unexpected directions.

(Awarding "High Risk" Biomedical Research behavior that intentionally creates "breakthrough infections" means "High Risk" in any direction and the freedom to unleash genetically engineered pathogens to create more "high risk" populations and discrimination is inviting even more emerging and re-emerging diseases already caused by the hand of science being rewarded in unexpected directions. Underexplored issues when breakthrough infections are likely to occur and Preparing Now To Assure Access to AIDS Vaccines For The World and prepare for Phase III clinical trials involving tens of thousands of volunteers and Of Monkeys and Men is the Bush Administration and co-sponsors preparing to nurture "breakthrough infections", as well as their lies to emerge and re-emerge disease and discrimination where the infections are likely to occur among the communities targeted to be controlled on many levels. The breakthrough infections have been well explored, but are swept under the rug because the Bush Administration has agendas for their infections (including the Avian Flu Virus, SARS and West Nile Virus), and as long as the hateful agendas are allowed to continue "breakthrough infections" will occur more and more often to more and more people. A priority for NIH and NIAID is recruiting minorities into clinical trials and to ensure that research results will apply to all populations affected by HIV as "high risk" is the biased and discriminatory nature of the Bush Administration whose top priority is to recruit minorities into the lethal clinical trials and then turn around and say behaviors of minorities is for everyone to notice discrimination void of accountability. What we need is breakthrough truth and not AIDS and/or related emerging diseases in AIDS or obstruction of justice or destruction of the truth or disaster or security issues or strategies and deceit all wrapped in a bundle, but peace without the political monster of the Bush Administration tied to a stone in a cave unable to emerge or re-emerge the truth ever or again.

The vaccine induced breakthrough infections and emerging diseases targeted to create community based alarm turns communities upside down and finding peace in disease is not likely to occur. A foundation of truth is required for a true a healing source to nourish that can turn the tide against those that are determined to hate "others" or "special populations" never to see the true beauty of personal struggle to emanate and populate forgiveness and love. The Bush Administration along with the pharmaceutical industry and the "Vaccine Enterprise" are gearing up to innoculate most of the world's population with lethal vaccines that are comprised of viruses, bacteria, chemicals, as well as insect and animal cells to propel their agendas of a new world control in order to order tomorrow. The breakthrough infections that are likely to occur in trial sites despite the prevention resources offered to the volunteers is saying that so-called safe behavior practices that are preached during the clinical trials will have no affect on the outcomes of the intentional infections that cause diseases in the targeted populations in the first place being enrolled in the lethal clinical trials, and the so-called "Phase III" clinical trials that involve thousands of volunteers. The breakthrough infections are everywhere there is even one new infection of HIV since it is the same basis of transmission via vacccines and medicine and not about safety of the vaccine or about human sexual behaviors. HIV transmission is about bad people abusing the masses one by one moving towards thousands of people at one time after another being blanketed with disease in breakthrough clinical trials involving thousands of innocent volunteers with no plans of ever making the cure acccessible.)

The Report titled;
    "2004-2008 Strategic Plan:
            Challenges and Critical Choices"
            U.S. Department of Health and Human Services
            National Institutes of Health
            National Center for Research Resources
            Bethesda, MD 20892-4874

http://www.ncrr.nih.gov/about_ncrr/StrategicPlan2004-08.asp

Says;

With increased use of "cyberspacebased" communications, investigators need access to more sophisticated computational resources for modeling, simulation, and data management.

As research becomes more multidisciplinary and team based, the research infrastructure must change. A different approach or paradigm must be used to train young investigators, and all members of the research team must receive credit for their respective contributions, especially junior investigators.

NCRR will address these and other emerging trends, as described in the goals and objectives set forth in the 2004-2008 Strategic Plan Many of the trends identified by participants at the Strategic Planning Forum were extensions of the trends noted in NCRR's prior strategic planning process. Respondents noted dominant trends in biomedical science such as: As genomes of species are fully sequenced, a greater number of genes are studied in mutant organisms, creating a rapidly expanding need for biological repositories and more efficient technologies to generate genetically altered models of human disease.

(As genomes of more species are fully sequenced, a greater number of genes are studied in mutant organisms, creating a rapidly expanding need for biological repositories and more efficient technologies to generate genetically altered models of human disease is heterogeneic separation of the human race with genocide and gene altercation to segregate special populations by physical attributes and disease to "dominate" "biomedical science" to dominate the world hidden in fluff of ambiguity of scientific emerging trends emerging diseases by the Bush Administration and company. The mutant mice, NIH mini-pigs, and the simian primate research center are just a few examples of the laboratory nightmares the government and certain industry monsters are creating in cross-species disease under the mad helm science of the Bush Administration using species as mere stepping stones to create human disease and a virtual biological warfare against humanity to gain control of the world. The vaccines and medicines of pathogenic viruses with hidden mutated species cells will create mutated humans species in time and obliterate peace of mind and trust forever in all humans cowering on all fours walking on eggshells. When will the madness stop?

(The genome project is being misused with designs to control people and behavior. If the government can find the elusive "gay gene" for example, or gene related to behavior or sexual behavior you can bet the Bush Administration will introduce the new technology into the human race. The Bush Administration and the Vaccine Enterprise are already altering genes to spread viruses not only between humans, but between other species and back to humans, as well as, culturing the viruses so antibiotics are not effective, and coding the viruses into the human genome to arise in infection at a later date. These disease spreading right winged nuts are hate mongers applying fundamental concepts of despise by using biological scientists to abuse and pass along the torture trade into humanity. The Bush Administration and the rest of the immoral majorities are constantly trying to find ways to alter natural human behavior in their usual abnormal belligerent behavior to create a superiority mess. The Bush Administration and company are looking for homologues in other species in designs at subtly altering the human species by way of heterogenic altercation and at the same time rewarded themselves financially in a twisted superiority complex of control similar to Adolph Hitler in Nazi Germany history.)

Again at the report titled;
Panel Session I: Cross-Species Transmission – Species Specificity and Tropism http://www.niaid.nih.gov/dait/cross-species/page3.htm

Says;

The porcine endogenous virus envelope does confer the ability to infect human cells, but it is not very efficient.

A significant cross-species jump occurred with adenovirus 76. Adenovirus 76 is normally found in ducks, but contaminated a manmade chicken vaccine and killed hundreds of millions of chickens. The virus is now established as a chicken-to-chicken infection.

Researchers are beginning to assess pig viruses for pig into human viral transmission. A porcine kidney cell line PK15 releases C type viral particles that can infect pig testes, ST-IOWA cells, mink cells, and human 293 cells. However, most other human cells are not infected. Yet, cocultivation with irradiated PK15 cells led to infection of a greater number of human cell types.

These PBMCs were co-cultivated with human 239 cells and ST-IOWA cells after the 5-day period. Both cell types showed increasing RT activity after a lag period between 20 and 40 days as well as a productive infection that spread efficiently. Thus it has been shown that infectious retrovirus can be isolated from at least two separate strains of the NIH mini-pig by mere mitogenic stimulation of PBMCs. Virus released from these activated cells directly infected both pig and human embryonic kidney cells.

It is possible that genetically modified pigs would be more capable of cross-species viral transmission and aborgation of hyperacute rejection will make pig envelope viruses more resistant to inactivation by human complement with some viruses being possibly pre-adapted for transfer to humans.

The overall picture indicates that retroviruses present in donor pig herds will be expressed in transplant tissue. It also seems likely that the recipient will become infected, particularly with immunosuppression to prevent organ rejection;; the immunosuppression will allow the virus to evade human immune responses. Currently, the key issues appear to be whether infection leads to high levels of viral replication in the transplant recipient and, if so, whether pathology results. Infection will most probably occur without associated pathology. However, infections could result in pathology that manifests many years after the transplant; some may give rise to cancers.

The Merriam-Websters's Medical Desk Dictionary Revised Edition definition of xenotransplantation; "transplantation or an organ, tissue, or cells between two different species (as a human and a domestic swine)"

(The mad scientists are designing genetically altered animals such as the NIH mini-pig and so-called knock out animals. The researchers are exploring ways to infect and affect humans and animals in an ever-growing arsenal of strategies of population control via targeting to demise. The mad scientists have genetically modified pigs so the genetically altered animals would be more capable of cross-species viral transmission as well as enabling pig envelope viruses more resistant to inactivation by human complement. In fact, some viruses are being pre-adapted for transfer to humans by the government using genetically modified animals to cause viral transmission in targeted humans to be labeled knock-outs. Some of the retroviral vectors produced in mouse or dog packaging cell lines are complement-inactivated when introduced in vivo as mentioned in the article and says the inactivation occurs by the exact same mechanism that causes hyperacute rejection in xenotransplantation. The government and co-sponsors are intentionally producing retroviral vectors in species cell lines to trigger a "mechanism" that causes tissue rejection or autoimmunity in "vivo" in humans oftentimes referred to as HIV/AIDS. The retroviruses present in the genetically altered donor pig herds will be expressed in transplant tissue and it is likely the recipient will become infected. The donor pigs are the governmental genetically engineered or "modified pigs" or "knock-out pigs" are more capable of cross-species viral transmission on purpose being used for viral coss-species infections.

The Adenovirus 76 is normally found in ducks, yet conveniently contaminated a manmade chicken vaccine and killed hundreds of millions of chickens. The virus is now established as a chicken-to-chicken infection exemplifies the intentional manifestation of a lethal vaccine made in a laboratory using a virus usually found in ducks to infect chickens not by mistake in order to give the world the illusion of viruses running rampant killing millions of chickens when in fact it was a manmade situation and happens to humans with HIV/AIDS. The sad part is the Bush Administration and the "Vaccine Enterprise" are using viruses harvested and/or genetically engineered in laboratories that have killed millions of people.)

A report titled;
"2004-2008 Strategic Plan:
Challenges and Critical Choices"
U.S. Department of Health and Human Services
National Institutes of HealthNational Center for Research Resources Bethesda, MD 20892-4874

http://www.ncrr.nih.gov/about_ncrr/StrategicPlan2004-08.asp

"Nonhuman Models for Biomedical Research"

Mutant Mice in High Demand
The mouse is one of the most commonly used research models to study human disease processes. It is small, easy to handle, and breeds rapidly. In the 1990s, researchers developed a method to create "knockout" mice; that technique selectively disables one or more genes and has created thousands of valuable new mouse models. However, researchers who create these unique, genetically altered animals often lack the facilities or staff to maintain and distribute the mice to other scientists.

More than 10 years ago, NCRR initiated support for a national resource for mouse genetic mutants at the Jackson Laboratory. However, the number of genetically altered rodents has expanded considerably with the sequencing of several dozen genomes. To accommodate this need, NCRR established the Mutant Mouse Regional Resource Centers. Created in 2001, the program consists of four regional centers and a central facility that processes animal submissions and orders from researchers.

Establish resources and improve the techniques for characterizing, standardizing, and cryopreserving important animal models, including gametes and embryos. Such technology is available for mice and zebrafish and should be developed for other animals, particularly non-human primates. The quality of animal-model characterization varies greatly across institutions, and only a few facilities are highly successful at freezing and storing viable embryos.

Increase the number of nonhuman primates available for biomedical research, and evaluate other methods to address the shortage of nonhuman primates. The need for these animals has risen substantially and is expected to escalate even more due to their essential role in biodefense, gene transfer research, and the increased risk of transmission of infectious agents to air travelers from remote areas around the globe.

Important animals alongside genetically altered and "mutant" animals that are more important in altering the human race is a real future up in the air and not grounded but slowly being altered to embrace only certain politically empowered humans embracing only a few human beings that are innately ugly in discrimination and not important human animals whatsoever. The current conservative political agenda twisted in sterile domestication to control qualifying or disqualifying life of diversity in true democracy is America wanning and turning upside down into a dictatorship of glorified inequality that has true grave consequences.

The design teams hiding in ignorance and apathy to manipulate and label human bodies as traits to be genetically altered palatable by a few is complete egotism wrapped in arrogance. The Bush Administration and company's pace of human destruction with controlled design researchers as mice spinning around in centrifuge labs around the world growing in deadly science silently overnight attending to plans for all animals and primates to be rank in file of importance genetically altered to be on the discriminatory list defying nature is cruel and unusual. Growing discrimination one by one to be unimportant animals unlawfully judged and abused by hate crimes for the future tense with worker bees as slaves and repercussions of whatever the political instigators see fit to be terminally ill is science and politics melding in evil concurrently ruling with intensity ugly intent stops dead the truth in Silence = Death. We need to put a stop to the Bush Administration and company's evil before their silent auction of humans turns into unstoppable rule altering our natural genetics to "knock-out" God from our spiritual planet inside each and every human being.)

Etiologic Agent Import Permit Program
http://www.cdc.gov/od/eaipp/

Says;

Etiologic agents, vectors, and materials containing etiologic agents are recognized as hazardous materials. Materials containing etiologic agents are regularly transported from one location to another by common land and air carriers.

The export of a wide variety of etiologic agents of human, plant, and animal diseases may require a license from the Department of Commerce.

HIV went from being maintained primarily, if not exclusively, in sooty mangebeys (HIV-2) and chimpanzees (HIV-1) (1-3) to being the etiologic agent of a worldwide pandemic. AIDS was not recognized as a specific disease until 1980, and HIV was not identified as the etiologic agent until 1983. Nevertheless, an estimated 16 million persons have died from AIDS worldwide with 50 million currently infected with HIV.

Etiologic agents are those microorganisms and microbial toxins that cause disease in humans and include bacteria, bacterial toxins, viruses, fungi, rickettsiae, protozoans, and parasites. These disease-causing microorganisms may also be referred to as infectious agents.

Any animal known or suspected of being infected with an organism capable of causing disease in humans may require a permit issued by CDC.

HIV exhibits considerable evolutionary potential and, with drug-resistant bacteria, may have done more to enhance widespread understanding of the importance of population and evolutionary biology to human health and medicine than any other example this past century.

Although HIV was initially susceptible to a variety of drugs, resistance mutations have enabled the virus to skirt every drug in the biotech arsenal.

The National Institute Allergy and Infectious Diseases Division of Aquired Immunodeficiancy Syndrome (DAIDS) mission statement located at www.niaid.nih.gov/daids/daidsover.htm

Says;

Issues have been raised with DNA vaccines; Part of the production process of DNA plasmids involves selection of bacterial cells carrying the plasmid. This selection is accomplished by culturing the cells in the presence of an antibiotic to which resistance is conferred by a gene in the plasmid. concern has been raised that resistance to the same antibiotic might be introduced in participants when the plasmid is used in clinical trials. Two precautions make this outcome unlikely. First, the antibiotic resistance genes contained by vaccine plasmids are driven by a bacterial origin of replication sequence (not a mammalian one) and are therefore expressed only in bacteria, not in host cells. Second, the antibiotic resistance employed does not involve antibiotics commonly used to treat human infections.

TheDivision's basic research efforts have yielded significant scientific information about HIV. For example, in recent years, DAIDS - funded investigators have identified new structures for viral components of HIV, additional chemokine co-receptors, and the existence of multiple, persistent HIV reservoirs even with the use of highly active antiretroviral therapy (HAART).

A report titled
CDC-FUNDED STUDY TO EXAMINE CRITICAL QUES-
TIONS IN HIV VACCINE RESEARCH April 2001
www.cdc.gov/hiv/vaccine/vislaunchupd-3-30-2.pdf

Says;

Drug Resistance – Researchers will also examine drug resistance in
those trial participants who become infected and enter treatment during the course of the trial. The agency will obtain blood samples from
all participants at the six sites who become infected during the trial to
evaluate the HIV strains for resistance to various HIV treatments.

The HVTN Pipeline Project located at www.hvtn.org of The National Institute of Health and the U.S. Department of Defense and at
the web page within the hvtn website located at
http://chi.ucsf.edu/vaccines/vaccines?page=vc-01-01

Says;

DNA vaccines are usually circular plasmids that include a gene
encoding the target antigen (or antigens) under the transcriptional
control of a promoter region active in human cells. The coding region of the inserted gene is followed by transcription termination and
polyadenylation sequences. To permit selection of plasmid-containing
bacteria during the production process, the plasmid also contains an
antibiotic resistance gene with a bacterial origin of replication. DNA is
generally less costly to produce than peptide or protein vaccines, and is
chemically stable under a variety of conditions. DNA vaccines are generally administered intramuscularly, using either a needle and syringe
or a needle-free injector.

The Report titled
"The current Status of HIV-1 Vaccine Development, 2004: Recomendations for the Future by The NIAID AIDS Vaccine Research
Working Group"
www.niaid.nih.gov/daids/vaccine/pdf/AVRWG/finalreport.pdf

Says;

Encourage development of a Human Challenge Model of HIV-1, wherein HIV-1+ patients on HAART would be vaccinated with more promising experimental immunogens. If they then elect to stop receiving therapy, the ability of the vaccine-induced immune responses to prevent, delay or modify the subsequent increase in plasma viremia could be a useful way to gauge vaccine potency." However, it must be noted that this experimental system is likely to be a more stringent test of the potency of a vaccine, because of the possibility that the pre-existing HIV-1 infection has already caused a significant level of immune impairment in the volunteers, despite their recent therapy. A mechanism would need to be found to provide the drugs for such a trial.

The Merriam-Webster's Medical Desk Dictionary definition of viremia the presence of virus in the blood of a host

(Once again more vaccinations with viruses as a guise of inducing an immune response with subsequent increase in plasma viremia is pure torture. To add insult to injury there is an evil twist to the above trial vaccinating already infected individuals with more viruses as a way of coercing the volunteers to stop taking their anti-viral medications that could be useful if the lab virus has not been rendered completely resistant to drug therapy. The Bush Administration is trying to find a mechanism to provide the drugs for such a trial to pivot into different drugs that are damaging to be in alignment with vaccine potency without resuming HAART therapy for the volunteers so once the trial is completed and the volunteer may not elect to resume potentially life saving HAART. The intentional damage and subsequent life threatening illnesses to follow designated a successful trial whether or not HAART is tainted to be worthless. The intense hatred towards the "Human Challenge Model" is to escalate the onset of life threatening challenges is apparent, but the twisted minds that are constantly dreaming up new ways to torture to speed up the process is a scary situation. The bad doctors that search for HIV in the blood after both HIV test showed negative to antibodies and bad dentists, as well as bad government and industry are infiltrating and destroying human life.

The amount of current bad doctors or dentists to infect the amount of people in the target populations to coincide with the Bush Administration Vaccine and Medicine Enterprise agendas of power, population and behavior control, does not compare to their agendas of global vaccinations and tainted medicines and manipulations that will enable the bush administration and the Vaccine and Medicine Enterprise to expedite efficiently their goals.)

Propagation of Primary HIV-1 Isolates www.aidsreagent.org/pdf-docs/virus.pdf

Says;

VIRUS EXPANSION CULTURE PROTOCOL

The procedure described here represents one method to prepare infectious HIV-1 virus stocks.

Positive growth of HIV-1 is detected by the appearance of p24 gag protein in the culture supernatant. The described procedure is employed by laboratory scientists, or others working in that capacity, to establish virus stocks of HIV isolate(s) by infection of PHA-stimulated normal donor PBMC with clarified infectious culture supernatant.

Reagent Preparation
Prepare all media/stock solutions at room temperature in a Class II biological safety cabinet. Unless otherwise stated, aseptic techniques should be used. Co-culture Medium Freeze Medium RPMI 1640 supplemented with: Fetal bovine serum, heat-inactivated at 56°C 15% Il-2 20 Units/ml. (IL-2 is available from the AIDS Reagent Program or may be purchased from a commercial source. L-Glutamine 2 mM Polybrene 2 µg/ml, prepared from 500 µg/ml Polybrene Stock Solution (page 3) Penicillin 100 Units/ml Streptomycin 100 µg/ml Combine the above components and filter sterilize using a 0.45 µ filtration unit. Label as "Co-culture Medium" with date prepared and expiration date. Store at 4°C ± 2°C. Discard after 10 days. The number of cells infected depends on the desired final volume of virus stock. For every 100 ml

supernatant 40 x 106 cells are infected. This type of expansion can be completed by using a one or two cycle infection process and this should be determined by the study director based on the availability and quality of virus inoculum.

(Not only are the "serious pathogens" genetically engineered and part of the vaccines and medicines, but they have also been cultured in the lab to be "antibotic resistant", as well as adjuvanted and boosted with additional vaccinations to integrate into human cells. First, why even culture and confer a bacteria to be antibiotic resistant to any antibiotics? Second, the government will not share medical records with doctors, especially if they are "good" doctors, therefore if the volunteer is infected with a virus that has been antibiotic cultured to be resistant to antibiotics after being in a clinical trial then the prescribed antibiotics would be worthless on purpose. "The antibiotic resistance employment does not involve antibiotics commonly used to treat human infections" is a lie since "penicillin" and "streptomycin" are mainstream antibiotics to treat "human infections." Another bold faced lie of the bush administration and the Vaccine and Medicine Enterprise creating "Autoimmunity" or AIDS and "insertional mutagenesis" of human cells causing cancer in unsuspecting innocent volunteers.)

The National Institutes of Health Fiscal Year 2003 Plan For HIV-Related Research www.oar.nih.gov/public/pubs/fy2003/iii_etiology.pdf

ETIOLOGY AND PATHOGENESIS
NIH Fiscal Year 2003 Plan for HIV-Related Research

Says;

The influence of new antiretroviral therapies, which are able to lower viral load to undetectable levels, on the natural history of AIDS is providing an unprecedented opportunity to gain insights into the pathogenic mechanisms underlying the disease manifestations associated with HIV infection and AIDS. Unfortunately, use of these therapies also is associated with a series of side effects and complications that we are just starting to appreciate and study.

Although the incidence of wasting has declined, it remains one of the most devastating aspects and one of the major causes of morbidity and mortality in HIV-infected individuals who do not respond or lack access to potent antiretroviral therapies, an issue in the developing countries.

However, since multiple concurrent causes of liver damage are associated with HIV infection including hepatitis viruses coinfection, antiretroviral hepatotoxicities, Ois, and cancers, the impact of each cause of liver injury on a patient's survival in an era of effective therapies is unclear.

Epidemiological studies in large cohorts will be instrumental in identifying changes in the causes of morbidity and mortality as a result of the availability of effective therapies in HIV-infected communities and in providing us with useful insights into their etiologies.

NIH supports a number of epidemiologic cohort studies focused specifically on women, adolescents, and children. The study of patient samples and of data generated by these cohorts is providing critical information about the mechanisms of transmission, the course of disease progression, and response to therapy in these populations.

A report titled Interpretation and Use of the Western Blot Assay for Serodiagnosis of Human Immunodeficiency Virus Type 1 Infections at
www.cdc.gov/mmwr/preview/mmwrhtml/00001431.htm

Because of the variability of unlicensed reagents, laboratories using non-FDA-licensed Western blots should compare, on a routine basis, their tests with the FDA-licensed Western blot kit using well-characterized serum specimens.

Although the overall sensitivity and specificity of the Western blot for detection of antibodies to the various viral proteins are high, there has been substantial debate regarding the interpretive criteria.

Furthermore, different Western blots (commercial, as well as "in-house"

preparations) and different virus-antigen preparations used to prepare Western blots may contain different numbers and concentrations of both viral-specific and contaminating cellular proteins that may have unpredictable molecular weights.

(It is all about behavior, and is a person is judged not to be in alliance with the bigoted ideals of government and industry then they will be attacked with viral agents. And the new emerging diseases such as West Nile Virus and Sars may have began as "in-house" preparations and now they are being distributed by government and industry in the same manner as the reagents called HIV/AIDS.)

The Report
NIH Fiscal Year 2007 Plan for HIV-Related Research
www.nih.gov

Says;

Fortunately, more organizations and companies are involved in HIV vaccines than ever before, and issues of coordination and cooperation have become an important component of the HIV vaccine agenda. The cross-agency Partnerships for AIDS Vaccine Evaluation (PAVE), involving key U.S. government agencies conducting HIV vaccine trials, led by the National Institute of Allergy and Infectious Diseases (NIAID), has developed timely initiatives for harmonization and coordination of selected aspects of HIV vaccine trials and their evaluation. This has led to close collaborations between Government sponsored trial sites and other networks and effected early implementation of some of the goals of the Global HIV/AIDS Vaccine Enterprise (GHAVE). In 2005 the NIH will fund the first of the vaccine centers imagined in the GHAVE plan.

A report
Promoting a Culture of Safety
www.ncbi.nlm.gov
Says;

Helmreich defines culture as a complex framework of national or-
ganizational and professional attitudes and values within which groups
and individuals function.

Corporate culture is often referred to as the glue that holds an organization together and is therefore assumed to be a contributor to or-
ganizational performance by socializing workers in a way that increases
commitment to the goals of the entity. It embodies a philosophy of
executive people that translate into and affects the behaviors of employees. The power of culture often goes unrecognized since employees may assume that the dominant paradigm is simply the way we do
things here. Regardless of the underlying theory health care is vulnerable to error. The application of safety promotion theories utilized to
positive effect in other high hazard organizations are being considered
for health care where accidents tend to occur one person at a time
instead of in sweeping disasters. Sagan uncovers a surprising amount
of evidence that also seems to confirm the Normal Accident Theory.
Three Mile Island nuclear accident was a Normal Accident Theory. As
a result, the term High Reliability Organization has been coined to
describe organizations with exemplary track records of safety; aviation,
chemical manufacturing, shipping nuclear power and the military.

(Indians send up prayers for nature to be a life force not a force to
be reckoned with and destroy spirit by a "dominate paradigm" of deceit
of freedom not informing "employees" that the "dominant paradigm"
in living life is simply the way we do things here on planet earth of no
votes counted and for all corporate behaviors to be inclusive of private
lives 24/7 to change into mold. HIV/AIDS and the laboratory generated "firm hand virus" during the Regan years was the beginning to
the invasive intrusiveness of the Patriot Act today in alignment with
the corporate co-sponsored world transporting viruses ear tagged for
HIV/AIDS labeling to be the dominate domain of how American does

things here on planet earth. Freedom being blind-sided by a dominate paradigm of the Bush Administration and co-sponsors abusing the Patriot Act by following "employees" into their private lives in America is a slow digression of freedom of spirit in America supposed land of the free with American history depicting Indians implanted into nature called "badlands" for affect. Disrespectful degrading purposes of labeling nature to be spiritually forgotten is the diabolical nature of the HIV/AIDS charade.

In Tampa Fl. For example city employees are not allowed to attend a Gay Pride parade or City libraries in Tampa are not allowed to rent books pertaining to Gay pride or display a Gay Pride poster during Gay Pride month is by no accident living in a "dominate paradigm" theory of today of no reality. If that is a "power of culture" bending the law of nature to be labeled disenfranchised then being bent and frustrated is of no wonder trying to convey nature is not an accident and the power of energy of spirit being scattered in America with the ashes of friends and family lost to the normal governmental accidents everyday of HIV/AIDS the charade. A pure loss of time of time for a chance to live free without constant grief and with healing not to be Silence = Death in a library everywhere for Gods sake is not normalcy anywhere.

Behavior modifications by a power paradigm without a choice of a broken heart to be heard in what is living as an individual in America of sublime choices? There is no "safe culture" in America only a "safety of culture" of the Bush Administration type cowardly people distributing viruses under the radar political table shutting down living along with messages of death and dying on a poster everywhere. Safety of Culture upside down of so-called professional attitudes in a vial descending out of nowhere from corrupt government and corporate power executives into our arms and mouths to behave disabled while they continue to invade our private lives as individuals with hidden agendas of intrusiveness being corporate citizens living on somebody else's standard time 24/7 is preposterous living for everyone. With no libraries to learn where is a safe place to learn to play and pray is a dismal life to live in

America today a Bush Administration political monster eliminating life today.

The Bush Administration denouncing nature demanding obedience against nature is causing humanity to be a lost culture stale and heartless in freedom of expression never safe. America today under the Bush Administration and co-sponsors of death and dying is creating an environmental prison of despicable conditions by them twisting citizenship over powered by a dominate paradigm of no accountability against nature green always appearing happy is the type of education we could do without in wasted time shrouded in compromises. Culture to an Indian is freedom of more than one "Philosophy" to live in harmony with animals and nature all different in a multitude of Aztec formations of colors and hues in our own world of cultural communication trying to live normal without so-called "normal accidents" or defining abnormal Bush Administration nurturing an Avian flu threat of nuclear proportions.

There is a God and a spirit of love no matter how much the social environment beats us up in messages of unworthiness. The spirit moves and so should we, and the spirit of support and comfort is happiness in realizing God wants us to allow others to live and in a way God is grateful for our prayers and actions of truth on earth and good will is for everyone. There is great comfort in realizing that we are doing God's will in life and how can there be comfort found in the Bush Administration currently ruining this nation that not only realize their own lies, but realize their lies physically injure people. How can G. Bush Jr. say that he loves God when his spirit in presence with words is a lie? G. Bush Jr. spirit is void of the love of truth and that makes his presence void of true spirit. G. Bush Jr. is a false entity garnering lost energy day after day preaching the will of freedom that is another lie in recognizing only a concept and never the heart of truth. Nobody should deny the love of God because that is what moves us in spirit and we are only vessels to allow His will to love to shine and for a president to believe he is in control of our lives to govern intentionally shut out the light of the truth is a dying garden with plants and seeds never being able to be nourished. We live in a commercial and capitalistic world with pressure and requirements to perform and produce and produce to perform or their will be worldly consequences and that is insane. Who wants that type of pressure? We are not human commodities, but real people being abused. America is moving in a wrong direction. The ultimate suffers are not the ones that do not produce or perform, but the people on earth such as the Bush Administration that intentionally causes pain and suffering to others yet in reality the Bush Administration is suffering today with no clue or desire to walk in someone else's shoes.

Panel Session II: Cross-Species Transmission Mechanisms of Pathogen Adaptation www.vrc.nih.gov/dait/cross-species/pages6.htm

Says;

Birds that migrate north and south are more significant for influenza transmission than birds that migrate around the world

Disease controlled gives the birds freedom to fly around the world in any direction, but with a cost of disease gives the Gay birds flying north and south grounded as unforgiven apple pie in america and the world diseased allover the world.

In a forgiving world we could get to square one, but the entanglement of Gay, Color, Straight, Economic Status the words and the actions in a direction of good faith are unable to communicate Silence = Death. The hate mongers distributing disease in all directions is forced upon us to fight the entanglement out amongst ourselves and the pieces of the fight are just game chips that are able to fall where they may in the hate monger's deadly game of controlling people's lives. The consequences of their forced hate and separation are meaningless to the evil pigs yet documented by them to perpetuate and grow their evil momentum in time and environment without a vision of peace. What is treatment? A facility? A day at the spa? Treatment needs equality first and then the people will follow in trust. Protect the birds and the tiny chirps of voices first in treatment and then war would be viewed at a different angle for everyone in the man made prison of government intrusion and death and dying. The governmental traps are the mind erasers of the ignorance that is determined to destroy anything that resembles the truth. The deceased AIDS victims had a lot to say, but were denied a voice and still we are unable to fly freely in voice of north, south, east or west.

The times spent or the times sent are an entanglement of hate and love. If we can not spend our time together sending messages of love in real production and creativity then the time spent is time spent and nothing else. Love does not grow out of thin air as money does on trees like carrots over our heads dangling in one big pinata with weapons at arms length away to burst open more time to waste. The entanglement of love in man made quick sand resounds unaware of the Titanic hitting ice as a mainstay of the loss in the political lost souls manning the ship in the wrong direction of life. Life to be on a ship of servitude to false political manipulators is unfruitful and boring as are the birds that fly around the world less susceptible to disease. Everyone that flies around the world wants more fly time bought and sold in corruption of all levels of life and that is the problem of selfishness of the old birds of the Bush Administration and the new birds on the Titanic both traveling around the world in train wreck speed and plastic fashion without a clue to stop and smell the roses in real time to stop the diseasing of birds that fly north and south. Love of controversy needs healing to agree to disagree instead of compromises that secretly is underhandedly compromising our health just so worldly birds can remain clueless captive and disease free.

Life needs to be lived not time spent dissecting and layering judgment to put labels on stamps of disapproval or compromised approval. Love needs love not nets and gaps to nets to end malaria but to end HIV/AIDS is malaria in conformity of labels, viral disease and genetic engineering viruses combined nets to profits in life lost freeing up land space at such grave costs. Inspiration comes with life being free to love not weighted down by the Bush Administration's harassing strategies that cause harm and removes life not to have another inspirational day one life removed at a time from life realized dead to HIV/AIDS is anti-inspirational. The Bush Administration's game of triggers and manifesting forced compliance is the same game they play trying to deceive nature does not compute to living. Ending reactions of Gay by judging behaviors with viral disease to induce cruel gossip glossing over life with more cruel judgements is not the truth seen in innate reactions to their games and strategies destroying a walk in life not an AIDS walk in life after the fact of societal sicknesses.

The soul by pure slaughter and of many souls feeling the same pain of the Bush Administration's game is day after day the same pain of expressionless life unable to express the HIV/AIDS charade with facts and cruel figures to the soul needing explanations not more fear of the game of death and dying day after day. A point across or a word down on a crossword puzzle the Bush Administration refuses to accept responsibility for their HIV/AIDS charade deceiving life to be mad at others and not a guilty plea for their crimes against humanity. Come on please a cross to bare really. At what point do we get to get the point across no more violence please?

No more targeting or recruiting people with strategies to convey superiority of acceptance or boosting low morale with viruses in a needle and a syringe would be a start to equality. Nightmare America is the name of the game with Education outlets on campuses to recruit for war, sports, or corporate citizenship should be banned and more emphasis on acceptance to broaden horizons with faith in humanity giving cohesiveness energy as a tool for ingenuity and family business. Genetic engineering viruses mutating and separating with strategies of recruiting judgement into society separating more the masses into more sadness of few choices in life swallowed up and never had a chance to grow saddened and confused is corporate/government strategies stealing our identities . The more individuality the more expression the more happiness with more small businesses and sporting arenas of amateur or professional sport not of negative separatism for an option of positive health status in transparency.)

A report
2004-2008 Strategic Plan:
Challenges and Critical Choices
U.S. Department of Health and Human Services
National Institutes of Health
National Center for Research Resources
Bethesda, MD 20892-4874

http://www.ncrr.nih.gov/about_ncrr/StrategicPlan2004-08.asp

Says;

Pursue strategic alliances with NIH components, other Federal agencies, industry, foundations, and other interested groups to provide access to essential biomedical research resources.

Today's climate of financial constraints and limited resources encourages organizations with similar interests to collaborate to achieve their goals. Organizations often can accomplish tasks that are of mutual benefit and can do so cost effectively, especially if the undertaking can attain an economy of scale. NCRR also avoids duplication of efforts by collaborating with other NIH components.

The objectives are to identify and overcome the barriers to strategic alliances, and establish models for private-public partnerships. Barriers involve patents and intellectual property rights, material transfer agreements, and real and apparent conflicts of interest.

Encourage collaborations among NCRR funded research resource centers to capitalize on each other's unique capabilities to solve complex research queries. Consider consolidation of research resources that hold complementary technologies.

Work in partnership with Federal agencies to identify and overcome regulatory barriers to research.

Collaborate with other agencies to accelerate the process of bringing biotechnology products to market.

Provide access to nationally distributed research resources for both NIH intramural and extramural investigators and encourage collaborative studies when the undertaking is of mutual benefit.

(The Bush Administration is aligning themselves with corporations and countries that have a vested interest in bringing biotechnology products to market and believe they can mutually benefit by instigating disease and profiting from the "products" sold, as well as the communities and individuals being held captive by intrusion and reliance on American organizations, as well as other interested groups be it American or international for so-called support against a disease descended upon communities and individuals by labs genetically engineering pathogens in order for the organized alliance to slowly gain control over human and land real estate. Government and co-sponsors are trying to identify and overcome the barriers to strategic alliances, and establish models for private-public partnerships to manipulate barriers involving patents and intellectual property rights, material transfer agreements, and real and apparent conflicts of interest to control their one way street of a path of destruction. Entities working in partnership with Federal agencies to identify and overcome regulatory barriers to research is crap and exemplifies the corrupt nature of the Bush Administration eliminating any FDA type regulations of safety. Any entity partnering with the Bush Administration in order to overcome the checks and balances system of legislation that sees the real and apparent conflicts of interest again exemplifies the real and apparent danger of a bullying system the Bush Administration and co-sponsors of death and dying are trying to impose on human health and peace of mind. Let us align ourselves with enacting change instead of the current corrupt government of hate and money imposing human aquisitions in our lives to be raped of life. The concept of inducing epitopes specifically selected to induce immune responses in most of the world's population is a scary and dangerous concept yet it is being attempted to be done nonetheless by the Bush Administration and co-sponsors of disease distribution.

It is sad Broke Back Mountain the movie was portrayed as a love story between two cowboys in modern day with no adventure except violence today. The story was about desperation from the start to the end of trying to cope with the political hostilities of yet today of no adventure except violence. Sure the two cowboys loved each other, but that was not the story line. The story line was about HIV/AIDS in reality and castration of the body heart and soul from the very beginning of boyhood of both cowboys the same today of no adventure in the current political environment to feel comfortable setting up as an alternative family and not end finalized alone dead in a ditch or alone in an isolated trailer in and around a dirt road. There could be no trailer or sequel to Broke Back Mountain since the story ended without any wonder or adventure other than loneliness far from love and alone in desolation of boyhood remembrances witnessing a Gay man castrated dead alone in a dried up river bed. If that is a love story today then where is life's adventures as a sequel to memories alone of life past manslaughter denied love of life by castration?

Love is short lived today capsulized in snippets of years forgotten by political judgment on purpose of what life or love is today or yesterday under forbidden adventure other than war. The carnival is not the same today as gypsies ranting and raving before HIV/AIDS with song for hours not noticing hanging over the edge in time as today the guilt being reinvented from war eras to castrate life cruelly unnecessarily demanding don't ask don't tell for government right winged hate mongers singing demands in their battle him the Gay of the republic pronounced immoral to the moral of soldiers brainwashed behind the years.

Desperation to feel alone in desolation never should be found in a love story from the start alone up and down a mountain on a dirt road booted out of society by labels. However, desolation is better for many than selling a soul as the Bush Administration does countless days on end escalating the rampages of HIV/AIDS leaving a void not repairable by any standards alone on a war ravaged road. Desperation in time is a sequel of no more dead birds after another rotting without the communication today to wonder free after a lifetime of purposeful forgetfulness not listening to forget me not please only deaf politics emerging into society demanding don't ask don't tell Silence = Death. Is the future just one more day in the unforeseeable future of more desolate war? Feeling trapped is the worst case situation when the truth is available to be unfurled and live in true awareness of our surroundings. America is a wasteland of nothing but desperation and coping skills being forced by a Bush Administration political road unforeseeable covered by fog.

Why is there not education to fill us in on the inadequacies of the system to not waste time learning on our own to be alone with the terror living in the political atmosphere of HIV/AIDS distribution and Silence = Death? Instead of disease why not just row after row of people judged inadequate and mow us over with rapid fire bullets? Would that not be more cost effective and less painful for us the victims of no choice in the matter? What is "deep" to survive political whims? What is living anyway? America is a terrible place to live and die because America ignores bloody fences of Matthew Shepard style hate crimes on a slay Christmas style stopping to put up more bloody fences on a holiday. America carrying forward today the weight of spiritual awareness of HIV/AIDS ignored is nothing gained of a past or current lives together with past and present tense jitters today ignoring the ignorant HIV/AIDS awareness today of no sense whatsoever except being bombarded by unexplainable phantom grief from the past in daily snippets not found on an HIV/AIDS poster dead or alive? Where is healing love?

America is a twilight zone being escalated to twilight zone disease status with real mass destruction being caused by twisted violent agendas under the table today by the Bush Administration arrogant slaying style building bloody fences. Stupid politics with stupid conservative compromises with ceilings and fences and no living Art liberating to have justified living in America today red white and blue beyond bruises in a pit surrounded by fences and ceilings with no widespread love. Red on white symbolism depicted in seclusion poster Art of violations in blood is sad living in America of no expression or identity of freedom beyond war symbols of the heart unable to express repression of don't ask don't tell Silence = Death. Military America today combining with the Bush Administration perpetuating don't ask don't tell Silence = Death equates to more busted legs and hearts and arms all along the way squeezing around broken red white and blue everywhere valuable time being wasted in time of dead or alive time in a life of G. Bush Jr. mantras of expressionless real fear of Silence = Death.

Difficulties at trying to start a life of your own in America is virtually impossible in a land of corporate and government citizenship advertised in America controlling people by repressive harassing attrition by the Bush Administration endorsing under the table with fences around their offensive ceilings captivating abstinence with no wide spread love. Red on white and only one color of symbolism is not Art bound in controlled blood of the HIV/AIDS charade tainting an awful picture of the future. Symbols real today are far from liberating to ease the fear factors of the Bush Administration utilizing adverse twisted communication deployment of arrogance never imagining what life would be living in their own compromises in their own strategic consequences in their own four walls adversely polluting the environment with wide spread repercussions.

The Bush Administration is full of liars spreading repressive ideals by distributing disease and war perpetuating inside down side freedom repressed agitating more people creating more energy to deter their ideals of arrogance into mush the dog bites being abused by government corruption and corporate co-sponsors becoming more and more wide spread.

Political compromises of death and dying are real today revolving and spinning involving innocence being of little or no consequences of the ripple affect the Bush Administration and co-sponsors of the HIV/AIDS charade has on humanity. Fair game and chance offerings are different in time of the game today of evolution that should be equality of life in years not a game of chance offerings of genetical discrimination that short changes time and humanity to be a game unfulfilled today as nature of the environment being corrupted and mutating altercations of humanity by the Bush Administration genetically engineering disease distribution with no transparency in Silence = Death for a chance to fight back and heal. There are grounds to stand up for nature to climb for humanities everywhere we are blessed with nature's trees plants and animals for human humanity to combine in love of nature together more joy in abilities to enjoy equality of life together supporting more joy of fair game is not the hunt destroying natural evolution and nature is not a game to be abused. Natural evolution involves billions of years with trees of Art to look forward to ringing in life poignant realities opposing abrasive time consuming fear realities of today's political atmosphere cutting down life short in a future of dead on arrivals nature today to be a human wasteland.

The Bush Administration spreading disease and war is not fair in their flash in the pan forced evolution of HIV/AIDS upside down awareness with fear becoming more prevalent with each new HIV/AIDS drug combination in and out of the bedroom. In fact, disease and war are unrelenting in chance offerings and windows of opportunity today for the corrupt "me too" corporations creating more silence and death corrupting more people by war games of a chance in hell offerings of rigid behavior control in and out of a vial. The current political environment today is noncompliant and disrespectful of nature's environment pliable and enchanting and not disabled and not the least bit interested to climb around with the corporate ladder grovel people living in bedroom gated communities.

Transparency is vital for life to live more than fair to love outside of love of game spiteful destroying love of communication and relationships natural in nature. What happens when the money runs out more trap doors to twist communications to bring humanity to its knees by a war game? Imagination forced to imagine the possibilities today under the gamey Bush Administration is dauntingly unimaginable realizing life is a battle today. Human will is better spent in peace to imagine equality of nature all the time and energy being wasted. Equality of friends seeing the same crap of the Bush Administration in game against humanity is comforting realizing friendship even without direct communication to feel energy outside of the Bush Administration life in a bubble so far away living in and around their painful wedge destroying communications in valuable time to heal togetherness without time being manipulated to be forced evolution as an disenfranchised entity of don't ask don't tell being taught in the Military. The Bush Administration and co-sponsors of the HIV/AIDS charade are all about violence creating war, disease and poverty forcing Global Warming and evolution to be real mutatations. Violence being causative agents to disease, war and poverty elusive type cast in so many ways of living ramifications especially virus violence culminating in AIDS that alters our genes with less time more valuable to share to heal outside of the Bush Administration era of don't ask don't tell Silence = Death. Right winged political eras with no healing time in sight is wrong not to begin life reversing ending life in our midst for essential living healing naturally will end political evolution ending a "short life to live". Communications with friends as family not to be forgotten in past eras of better communications of love needs revitalization to diminish violence today under the Bush Administration of no communication era ending peace, prosperity and longevity. And love awareness of natural evolution needs to be cognative of longevity not to be ended again and again by discrimination politics that created HIV/AIDS in the first place ending our vision of a long life to live in love as nature intended not to be second to violent pollution.

The Bush Administration and co-sponsors of death and dying must be stopped to end violence permeating into humanity to voice a real difference of silence = death both debilitating to our psyche health and well being silent for too long. Healing love with death of loved ones to heal and stay afloat sometimes sad to be alive. Home is where the heart is in the Gay community not to be torn apart again and again never to grow old with lasting memories of love to savor anew for more time lasting in healthy time and not just time. Art as dance is beautiful of physical importance today to continue Art to dance everlasting is essential to love of life to live to end the battle of silence = death and disease labeled HIV/AIDS ending physical Art by shear discrimination. Problems and no apparent solutions levitating us astray to divorce life and live in America of little diversity causing disenfranchised to swelter in problems and waiting to live or die is the problems to our solutions unfortunately needing political compliance to end HIV/AIDS year after year for people to live better together to end disenfranchised living. Volunteers of a food drive for HIV/AIDS victims should be paid volunteers 365 days of the year for more awareness of HIV/AIDS for a better reach of awareness of why plight of disenfranchised is no volunteer to government disease. More healthy money needs to be available for the entire table of people living with HIV/AIDS and volunteers for all people affected physically and emotionally trying to live in comfort of a meaning to life in time to be healthy the best we can under the current conditions. Being a shut in to HIV/AIDS and hungry is never understood in silence yet HIV/AIDS awareness ravages 365 days of the year into the public to be upside down in caring disregarding the root of the problem of government and co-sponsors distributing disease.

It requires many voices to get to the truth and we must stand together before we can unveil the truth, and trust in each other that we can be heard and we can give. It is not brain surgery, it is faith in each other that gives us the strength to prevail. It is easy to hide from the repression whether it is a stay at home relationship or a job or whatever, but in reality we need to pull together as one to battle the monster head on because it is intensifying with strategies to disease. It is paramount we all get involved against the hidden agendas that are in the wings of the White House waiting to murder and further trample on the Gay community. We need to be seen as the healthy and viable community that we are and a party in life always trumps any party in politics. Just to have the freedom of speech and the right to expression without hate and judgement are simple avenues to happiness, yet the hate and judgement is ignorant to life and as a result we all suffer stuck in time. Time is stolen from us everyday under the bush administration and that is sad. My words are held captive on my computer since I am targeted with control and money issues that disable my ability to even print and convey my speech. America. I would love to share my words with the Gay community as a reversed AIDS awareness and have a sense that my time is not spent in vain. And by the way, hating my friends to hate me is despicable, yet a reality under the bush administration spending ignorantly time and money in a wasteland of control that has destroyed countless lives. Fuck when will it stop?

Gay has been around since the beginning of time and time being Gay in America under the evil pigs of control such as the right winged Bush Administration of conservative compassion is not a democracy but a hypocrisy of judgment that murders with disease out of spite of perception. America is not healthy when the so-called leaders believe their mission is to destroy the lives of others that have been perceived and judged in the past and adhere to those past bad perceptions instead of having the courage to realize the ignorance in perception when it involves demeaning and belittlement of fellow human beings and thus have the gumption to say no to the continuing abuse. However, life is far from fair and the ignorant evil pigs in power with a national treasury at their disposal believe Gay is not normal or even worthy of being on the same playing field, and as a result, we continue to be stuck in time in a compartment of judgement and perception where inflicting disease is the evil pig's answer to handing down judgement to their perceptions. Around and around they go and where will anyone be in five years let alone another generation from now if the death and dying and false perceptions and Avian flu and HIV/AIDS cycle is not eliminated?

The continuance and stepped up basis of the Bush Administration's HIV/AIDS charade has amplified the ill-conceived perceptions, stigmas, and judgements, and as a result, has broadened and intensified the overall misconception around the world regarding the Gay community and is that normal? The evil pigs stamp a label of hate on the Gay community and in addition they publicize their hateful perceptions as deviant behaviors of innocent bystanders that require intervention of disease because of perceived behaviors. We can not even get past a fucking behavior and focus on the real crimes stemming out of perceptions and reactions to harmless behaviors that have put many of us in the ground. Fuck, if we were to get back to basics Gay would not even be relevant. We need to re-educate our hearts to accept that are we are who we are and nobody behaves normaly. What is normal? How much more do we have to endure before the murdering stops? Gaps in time are for the ignorant in control that have nothing better to do with their time than to keep us separated in gaps of perceptions that disables the truth. We are always kept at arms length away from each other and the truth.

The compliant behavior card to disease should not be played any longer just to get along in a world that has best interests in normalcy to gossip. Advocacy is just a word under the evil pigs of control of democracy, but in reality it is advocacy that gives life to democracy in real time if only the control element were not part of the equation to be an advocate for ending HIV/AIDS. The control paradigm of the evil pigs include their fear of the truth being revealed and thereby destroys the advocate in all of us that have a voice beyond the occasional vote at the polls. Why wait for new measures to be put on the ballot that rarely have substance to magically appear when the real measures and issues will never be on any ballot magically or otherwise because of the control that dims our hearts. Death and dying amongst the HIV/AIDS charade that has tentacles to encapsulate and trap the last of the advocates will be our demise. We are lying to ourselves if we truly believe that advocacy is healthy in America today in a way that reveals the truth not advocacy where the advocates are sold a bag of lies where the advocacy mutates over to the enemies side because of control. Real advocacy is yet another dying breed in America close to extinction. We will need to redefined our lives in order to compensate for the governmental lies that sour society and thus eat at our hearts while we realize the truth in silence, and subsequently living in mere existence.

The decades of lies have created a life form of bigotry and money over matter and the rulers of the lies cherish their nurtured monster that is unforgiving and programed without the truth as a money loving machine that only needs adjustments to account for the new human targets being gobbled up by new prejudices with the same "end result." When will real voices be heard with the preciousness of voice being held up in servitude and nurtured instead of being held up in silence in confinement reverberating off walls of injustice that are afraid of voice? Why do we want to silence the truth when the truth is all we have to save precious lives? The voices of real advocacy will fade under the current repression and regret will not be in the hearts of the few remaining voices of justice that are snuffed out by either control, disablement or death, but regret will haunt those that only listen and did nothing. Why is the world mute when it comes to life or death? We either accept each other as living human beings or we accept the perceptions that lead to misconceptions and judgmental lies that subsequently forces us to embrace premature death out of hate and spite created by the hands of a few individuals still perpetuating and nurturing their monster lie of HIV/AIDS. Eventually we will not even give the HIV/AIDS charade a second thought since it will be far too ingrained as "the way it should be" and getting to the root of the massive problem will be lost forever.

The Bush Administration can not even be a puppet since the strings fall out of their slimy membranes they advertise as a backbone without accountability. An amoeba has more fortitude than the Bush Administration that can not even stand up for humanity. A spineless wonder without wonder and a pack of lies up their ass is all that holds them up. Why do we have to be forced into submission of a bucket of crap. Every day validating our existence as a Gay community in the 21st Century is beyond believable times one two thousand seven and climbing out of the pit of lies of the Bush Administration in a comma should not be our responsibility. Accountability is not what the Bush Administration believes but a twist in strategy and control with money and viola accountability and responsibility is reversed and a double whammy is beset on the targets they hate namely the Gay community as morale and societal demise. Fuck, is it really even worth our while to even respond to such nonsense yet it is our lives they are manipulating. But why? Why must we climb into their world of intrusion when we want to heal, and better ourselves? Gay is not the enemy and the people that have nothing better to do than build tunnels of seclusion instead of bridges of love in the daylight will never be more than a pit full of doom and gloom. When will we be able to get along, in our lives to walk on a bridge of understanding that would be easy to build to the "outer world" if it were not for the noise of the deconstruction era of the Bush Administration? One step forward in humanity and two thousand steps back in time is the illusions of an administration that wants totalitarianism when totalitarianism is and never was, but just an illusion. We need to wake up America and realize our enemies are within since that is the game?

The Bush Administration has always been about death and dying and Gay and so-called minorities have been victims all along, and is that what we want? Is it even a fair game? It is just so fucking sad. Why do we have to validate? We validate only because of the hate every day. Around and around we go and the likes of the Bush Administration will not stop until the backbone of America becomes correct against their bent minds and we see that life is more than judgement and we experience an out of the shell awakening that would be embraced by all Americans regardless of our set ways or our brainwashed ideals that set us back because of HIV/AIDS over and over again back in time because of what? A sexual preference? A black TV channel? What? It is just so tiny how we live. Why does the sadness outweigh the good? We as a Gay community are not prideful in the "conservative" nonsense, but we are proud. Being proud is a communion of spirit and we as a Gay community are here for each other just as everyone could be on planet earth if love were allowed to communicate outside of the confines of Silence = Death. We love who we are, and just want to get along in a humane society. The governmental intrusions interrupt our ability to interact with the so-called moral majority a minority and if we are continually intentionally in abrupt mode of disconnect and consequentially in a state of flux in advertised hate and don't ask don't tell Silence = Death then how does society believe we can fend for ourselves to end laboratory HIV/AIDS of spiritually and emotionally drained?

The governmental lies that the Gay population is affluent is a lie and maybe 10% of the 10% publicized as being Gay are affluent, but that is and never should be the fucking issue. Just more publicized lies. The Gay community needs no more labels or statistics and all we need is the fucking truth. Priorities are not a business plan or daily chores. Priorities are to take care of ourselves as a community and by doing that we take care of each other and taking care of oneself does not mean money but being true to self is the best care one can give to one and all. In reality we have each other Gay, Straight, Black, Brown, Yellow,

White, Rich or Poor as a resource if America would stop judging. It is all just so fucking sad, the delineations we build around ourselves. Grievance money drains our human resources. The life insurance agent tabulates the amount of life insurance the company can offer by the current "standard of living" the individual is living and if the individual's worth or income is not at certain level then it reflects on the amount of life insurance offered and that is where we are in America. A standard or expected way of living just because of past and present experiences of having money is just so lame when the real actuaries are our friends and family that realize our true self worth. In the Gay world we are not even allowed to have intimacy of friends as family, and if we do, we jeopardize our lives by governmental inflicted disease and control that reverses the actuary tables on all levels of society. We should be compensated for the lives lost of our friends and family at the hands of government and the pharmaceutical industry as well as compensation for the individuals currently labeled as HIV positive and living with a man made disease under the control of government and the pharmaceutical industry that prioritizes behavior over life. And compensated for the abuse and loss of life because of same sex attraction coping and trying to cope with HIV/AIDS in our community testing our blood.

HIV/AIDS also requires healing emotionally and mentally to understand what happened to us being advertised lost when we have been here all along. Economics has not even begun to consider the human being in America or around the world. There was a time when advocacy really meant something, but HIV/AIDS was created as a revenge tool and a scare tactic that tried to prevent us from communicating, and advocacy has been set back to less is more in time. We as individuals that comprise the Gay community live to be true to ourselves and that alone enables us to be vigilant and strong against the Bush Administration that uses endless strategies and tactics that are ignorant and harmful of nature as a result we are advocates for each and every one of us together defying them the opportunity anymore to steal our bodies and hearts being true to ourselves with the truth of the HIV/AIDS charade in our minds.

The bush administration hates Gays, yet we are everywhere and as a result hate is where they draw their energy thereby the environment is disabled by an infrastructure of hate. The ignorance of hate designed against a community that lives to be true to ourselves and subsequently true to each other as an extension of self is probably the most vial form of hate destroying our nature is off limits to their culminating into physical harm being inflicted by an infrastructure of disease. The evil pigs of the Bush Administration and their advisories with their gadgets of surveillance and strategies to control is not intelligence. Intelligence comes from love, but the evil pigs living in a whirlwind of control by disease always searching for a windfall at the expense of others just to feel intelligent is not a part of natural living. The only windfall of substance is togetherness from heaven of the ones in love with humanity.

The Bush Administration concentrating on whose love to squeeze the life out of with the Gay flag to burn simultaneously to be demonstrative in subtle loud discrimination power struggles the Bush Administration. Diseases do not hold water in repertoire not able to send a greeting card because of health issues to farmlands anywhere in America being robbed of energy by disease because of deep arrogance the Bush Administration and co-sponsors harbors out of spite living in hate of a blue state or Gay sexual orientation or the myriad of Parents and Friends of Lesbians and Gays (PFLAG) living in red and blue states putting the Bush Administration to test in which they brought on themselves hate begets misdirected hate.

The Bush Administration and co-sponsors of the HIV/AIDS charade see power thru their mad red eyes hungry and evil starving for absolute power over people at any costs to catapult the HIV/AIDS charade living a power addiction over adverse reactions of humans suffering. The Bush Administration living an agenda of delusional values of themselves as "players" in their game as an opposing infrastructure of unavoidable Nazi style superior life in attempts to slate slanted to red state ruled on a dime creating more delusions in their minds to start an avalanche of corrosive conversion processes advertising abstinence living and population control as a "fitter family" of moral values wrapped in sterile seeds on a farm not for thought of a child living with

HIV/AIDS unable to send a greeting card. The cultural spirit dampening and dwindling and growing in numbers across America expressing less of the HIV/AIDS victims is becoming a wasteland more than a wasting syndrome of a human life blood warm red and with eyes to a soul to send a greeting card. The Bush Administration is pulling the wool over America's vision of the future not to be humane diverting attentions to affliction and not affection and to a life of war, disease and military control as they revel in their swift moves of sweeping the HIV/AIDS charade under the proverbial rug day after day across red and blue states and across oceans of tears. George Bush Jr. is a divider not a decider.

The living nightmare of the HIV/AIDS charade must not be allowed to continue. The cycle must be severed for the health and well being for everyone. We must begin the healing so we can move on with our lives instead of living in this nightmare the Bush Administration is creating and calling us their owned. We should be allowed to be free in America to live healthy and fruitful lives without dire consequences because of a "Gay lifestyle" or the color of our skin or rules of when to sing or when to voice Art in dance of how we should be serving the served. We are upside down in America and we should be striving to dance and sing all of the time to free up space to be joyful of more life not fearful of less life being offered by "superiors" valuing judgement confining expression out on a limb.

America does not understand sadness since sadness is a form of vulnerability against what? A fortitude of war? We better start understanding each other or sadness will always be a behind the scenes reality that can not be exposed because of the many wars on many fronts that will never end. We can learn from sadness so much that would leave war in the dust, yet our morals are a one-sided definition in America as a right to a life or dead or alive and we still cry in silence. America causes so much pain yet we stand tall for what? America is only vulnerable to the evil American right winged political pigs that causes so much pain and suffering creating bad will within the facade fortresses of "dead or alive" or "win at all costs" is tired news.

Why is war a game when sadness is not even exposed? The Bush Administration is playing the same old card game of America a young and new beginning when in reality we are full of illusions that never pan out because of the wars. A new beginning is saying no to war and meaning no more war with weapons or viral diseases internal or otherwise. America with bad leaders have gone astray and brainwashed into a barrel 'o bad with nothing to wear but illusions of shiny that is on the opposite side of the spectrum of joyful people of America today. The Bush Administration does not say for many and their actions are way worse than our beliefs, yet the typical American citizen seen by the "rest of the world" is a mess. It all comes down to trust and forgiveness, and we have lost both in America not to mention an all time record national deficit and HIV/AIDS related infections and deaths with a president saying the same old thing his daddy said "read my lips no more taxes" except for war and death tolls of war and disease.

The Bush Administration is all about corporate dollars and not family dollars. America better wise up or we will be corporate citizens or a mutated mess of diseased and genetic alterations with accompanying pharmaceutical servitude. The Bush Administration is angry over itself and not in a right place let alone a frame of mind that is understandable. The Bush Administration is so ignorant because the world is passing them bye that they can not even see straight, yet attack what they maniacally label as "bent" or "queer" or "fags." Why is validation of Gay an everyday occurrence in America? What do we have to prove? When will time overcome validation? The proof is in the facts, yet we are a recipe for politcal stance of circumstances of abuse being used and yet we give unconditionally to each other within a second and gladly over again time and time again being Gay all our lives.

Gay under the microscope is tired hat being politically infiltrated and abused and the recipe is in the genes. Being proud or our lives is only for the eyes of love that does not judge. The evil pigs are not welcome, and they are off limits to our true nature even if miracles do happen and then they would learn. We must separate from the abuse as a healthy step in the correct direction because of the horrendous abuse with unnecessary death and dying that is becoming a mainstay against the Gay community. We are good and many are tired of explaining ourselves just to survive. The microscope needs to be moved over to the other side where a microscope would on corruption of government and co-sponsors of flagrant abuse. Being put under the microscope in a sterile climate does not need validation since we have already validated our love to live and give. The hate mongers are the naive party that need removal so the abuse and harassment will end. Life under the repression of the Bush Administration is fourth world that abuses the system to label their targets as "naive" is once again a battle amongst themselves to feel superior and using human beings as scapegoats to achieve their inadequacies sprewading disease is nothing more than another abusive clinical trial, doctors visit or a dentist appointment. Being blind sided by departments of abuse with vaccines or vials of vial is not a definition of humanity being discriminated or hated, but a definition of the instigators being criminally insane. Being naive is a good thing under the correct microscope without all the prejudices and judgements from opaque minds that blur in one hand and all the vaccines, medicines and bad intentions that create disease in the other. The age of innocence being lost is forced by man. Naive is a good thing with or without a microscope, yet it is frowned upon by the hardened criminals that make fun of human frailties and in turn have no levity of spirit. They fall on their double edged sword every day with bad intentions out of spite and hate. Hate is never truthful. Love is the truth.

Companionship is different than marriage of sexist rules by "deciders" demanding one sided protection cut in half from the lives of people that do not even want anything to do with the right winged hate mongers intruding into our lives. What is more fair love or war? All is not fair in love and war today under a dishonest "decider" in the Bush Administration of more dishonest "deciders" that only protect themselves from themselves. Marriage of one man one woman is only the tip of the iceberg of the HIV/AIDS charade attacking labeled minorities calling us "high risk" disenfranchised vulnerable and diseased incapable of their "decider" marriage dividing a nation in a time of crisis of don't ask don't tell Silence = Death by viral bombs and war. In crisis of the HIV/AIDS charade we have learned to pull together finding love of real compassion turning away from dividing authority not divine that uses disease to modify behaviors and not the true nature of love or gestures of sincerity finding warmth and companionship in time trying to pull away from a Bush Administration war maze of strategies being installed into the environment of an HIV/AIDS theater of chaos physically advertising war and hatred. The HIV/AIDS infrastructure today of awareness and healing apparatuses being withheld in containment of don't ask don't tell Silence = Death being installed in the theater of awareness upside down is sad and needs desperate change to occur today. Healthy living requires awareness of compassion not compassionate conservative jargon putting guidelines on compassion dividing life of many people to be drafted without a choice into the HIV/AIDS charade of lethal drug and medicine administrations with no conservative compassion allowing more people to live.

Sexual harassment by the Bush Administration trying to modify behaviors that are not innate feelings, and as a result causing heartache and misery with no transparency and fear attrition strategies they use today is living life in a corner with no simplicity to be free to be Gay innate feelings being abused in a corner of Silence = Death.

The fewer transparent opportunities in America the more rip torn from cradle to grave told what to do every step of the way removing life slowly of molasses never to learn energy in fast moving happiness of togetherness as a whole. America lopsided by money staining the judges to dictate law into the hands of political opportunists of evil master plans strangle lives to be separated into professional slavery arenas is not happiness anywhere. America is a suffocating arena mauled with few opportunities to network together to be healthy ants farming not caring what human judge wants to spy with no life to make sure their culture is safely controlled. Removing life out of our midst to remove prayerful vision for each other together is the worst of the worst with the HIV/AIDS charade of no expression, no energy and no ingenuity of genetically engineered viruses made by opposing views of government scientists and researchers mentally ill and paranoid.

Life is stolen in America of no identity. America monopolized by money started with microsoft and America went into a tail spin. Bill

Gates painted a picture of rotten economics and only he and the right wing strategies could save America. Bill Gates is not new nor is the concept of monopoly, but rather more conservative action new in less diversity is better lost as so many do in time of self admiration of a job created by political business. Bill Gates and billions of dollars transposes overseas into billions of dollars in Malaria and AIDS growing uncontrolled and disguised as charity, but in reality it is more deadly deterrents to diversity and life and not awareness of the water of tears being trampled in time of nightmares in America monopolizing upon delusions to create more viruses causing more discrimination and violence. Bill Gates refuses to build a building of true respite or even an outlet for real food in their disease riddled areas, but more than willing to fund research venues and clinics under clinical conditions to distribute bacteria and viruses of decimation as cheap as possible. Even the mosquito nets for malaria Bill Gates alludes relief by walking around in the devastation are being provided by outside volunteer resources while the International AIDS Vaccine Initiative a business of the Bill and Melinda Gates Foundation continues ravaging lives in clinical settings.

The Bush Administration, Bill Gates and company refuse to see internally the spirit of the massive number of individuals being voided in falling tears on their foundation of blight building more and more clinics to open more and more doors to step into despair in need of real shelter of the human trauma being bestowed upon humanity. Instead, Bill Gates and G. Bush are caught shuffling the daily news to squirm around and slimly turn more capitol dollars given monopoly status into continuing the glorified money laundering viruses of despair on the underground drama train aiding the right wing master plan to control humans and human nature.

The Bill and Melinda Gates Foundation created several years ago the International AIDS Vaccine Initiative in which the foundation is continuing to heavily fund in laundered capitol monopoly money for IAVI to distribute the Vaccine Enterprise of distributing viruses and bacteria churned out from the National Institute of Health laboratories to add more diabolical genetics in a virus with a twist of business savvy of a job well done spreading disease. The business monopoly mind of disease distribution is a bad combination and should be destroyed under the despicable political business belt tightening and suffocating life. We need to protect our health if we are to sustain life, and during the process now we need to not capitalize on installing in our spirit ideals of crappy monopoly money being poured into a Bill Gates addiction of dirty business practices to bring us down in more ways than one with varying HIV/AIDS initiatives. Instead, we need to become aware of the business of health wrapped in politics and to put under a microscope a true analysis of what savvy means to the health of a person or to unscrupulous business practices in health care in a lethal Vaccine Initiative of more layers upon more and more viruses in syringes. Silence = Death and individuality with better ideas regarding life should never be destroyed by political ignorance battering in rhetoric conclusions of evidenced based lies and swimming in consequences of a twisted right to our lives using more money to deter the truth of equality. The new disease creations with genetic twists the Bush Administration and company concentrating efforts in generating designer labs as outlets around the world to encode more than just disease into vaccines and medicines to infect innocent people. The Bush Administration's new strategy as a business acting on initiatives within a master plan to gain population control as delusional power is just a vaccine away to be profound power over innocent individuals. Individuals lined up to be science projects and walk with disease as advertisements of fear will never end unless we are allowed to communicate.

The government and research experimentation schemes and business initiatives being enacted against individuals to be pseudo corporate citizens to "behave" with no choices whatsoever in life are schemes of infections controlling society as cultures in test tubes that isolate individuals and instill behavior controls and labels as signs of the times of business success in executive power. The HIV labels of various strains of viruses, bacteria, chemicals and genetically altered species cells are used to label people as HIV/AIDS disease in concluding behaviors to advertise consequences of behavior to create fear and freeze the masses. Corporate citizens with annoying "behavior traits" are not conducive to the don't ask don't tell power people enjoying a shower of money and greed in the business schemes recycling life as a constant "house cleaning" giving more land space complete with slavery to evil entities. The business of disease distribution to eliminate unwanted people as a business item in cold blood extractions from mother earth growing colder in oil burning real life is the real terrorism contained in Silence = Death as the proverbial enigma nobody wants to dissect.

This blatant attack to extract, target and infect selected individuals, communities and countries is genocide in the exploratory planning stages using war today, and pure real life torture in loss of innocence. If the devastation is allowed to continue life will not only equate to starting the day with an alarm, but all life will begin and end with many alarms of many more wars on the horizon. We as humans are part of the animal world trying to do the best we can, but unfortunately in the unnatural world of the Bush Administration and company we are fortunate if we can do anything under their control and forced demise trying the "best they can" to create difficulties and compromises of natural immunity. Life is difficult enough the way it is in America without the Bush Administration meddling destruction into our lives causing confusing and interruptions trying to be the best a person can be. What really is the best we can be, especially if ill with their disease, requested to don't ask don't tell or wounded in their many wars of Silence = Death? Many are fed up with the decimating crap of "Federation America" tearing US apart in more ways than one! How can anyone be the best under the reality of Silence = Death and don't ask don't tell if Gay as a lifetime in the closet? The heartache of internal silence is more than unhealthy it is abusive to tell people not to say a word about the HIV/AIDS charade. Hate begets hate with violence, and in fact, gender violence being subjective in America within the mantra prayer of "never hit a female" is a notion to imagine violence to culminate to physical abusive battering activities. Why hit anyone or dream of violence or tell someone they cannot defend themselves being glued to don't ask don't tell within the repugnance of America that is barbaric and uncivilized? Why allow America to be put into a military box? Why hit anyone within the "hardest hit" communities especially under the auspices of internal silences and sadness already rip torn unable to say defense out in the open for the best someone can be in Federated American war!

Federation America needs more social scorn on battering, and less on mantras of don't ask don't tell of the internal violence felt being battered and punished in the closet of HIV/AIDS surrounding the person feeling the bruises from the outside in. The closet in the military is viewed as an inanimate object to nourish, yet a person must be quiet on the inside? That is pure inequality to be the best anyone can be. Being Gay is not a crime and inequality disables our ability to grow and destroy the hate in the American air to transform towards acceptance on the natural tolerable ground! "Be All That You Can Be" only in military terms of "Be All The Military Wants You To Be" and no questions asked of substance or meaning so boring and not real is Federated America. Real gives more meaning to life than the current "America" under the Bush Administration giving real harassments for real grief especially in an natural setting creating deeper discontentment and greater heartache alone and disassembled.

America today is a terrible place to live and die being harassed from cradle to grave just for being Gay along with targeted with a manmade disease to "be all you can be" living in America today. The manmade agendas of the Bush Administration and company forcing people to be compromised more than an immune system in controlled behavior stigmas is torture. Military America constantly at war to be all a person can be or being all one can be harboring a manmade American disease called HIV/AIDS are the strategies being implemented to change the world's society to a society of one cement strip around the world controlled by borders, yet beyond any territories utterly being decimated and chipped away by control.

Discrimination today in Federated America is subtle on purpose and more intense because of the subtleness of Federated America targeting individuals deemed a person "ruining morale" within a special rights population of the military of inequality of "special forces" the world to change for the worse being manipulated without true freedom. Cemented in everywhere in infrastructure guiding our every move with a criminal Patriot Act invading our private morals does more destruction than showering with soap and a Gay person clean. Federated America moving US towards a slow death of individuality ill-judging with insane behavior corrections of disease and war bullying not to be so "different" after all is sad and done dismal in infrastructure leaning towards occupation of individuality to easily put people away into categories of limited choices. Basically, the Bush Administration and co=sponsors are creating a world prison complete with torture. The more young people being lost to military instruction or the wider scope of individuals lost to Federated Disease called HIV/AIDS within targeted neighborhoods, campuses or "special population" categories to be targeted the stronger Federated America becomes a stale and grotesque status quo.

The Bush Administration forces behavior control with cattle prods putting people into cattle yards surrounded by fences and no freedom is experienced in their environment of military disease distribution and less apt to have love change for good intentioned individuals alive to be creative and avoid war altogether. If "Federated America" is allowed to continue turning back the hands of time unchecked of the Bush Administration's harassments being bestowed upon humanity then eventually the only robustness in life will be bigger harassments in bigger cattle yards giving instructions to harass and target individuality with bigger cattle prods to be the norm for all time within military timing our zone to be forever interrupted. Federated America is directing towards deeper levels of "haves" and "have nots" with don't ask don't tell Silence = Death being a military secret only allowed for the "haves" to discuss behind closed doors. The continued harassments being left unnoticed in America says America is uncaring and many countries beyond Federated America already realize America is an arrogant uncaring place to live to never care for individuals judged outside the American military "status quo".

The Bush Administration forces behavior control with cattle prods putting people into cattle yards surrounded by fences and no freedom is experienced in their environment of military disease distribution and less apt to have love change for good intentioned individuals alive to be creative and avoid war altogether. If "Federated America" is allowed to continue turning back the hands of time unchecked of the Bush Administration's harassments being bestowed upon humanity then eventually the only robustness in life will be bigger harassments in bigger cattle yards giving instructions to harass and target individuality with bigger cattle prods to be the norm for all time within military timing our zone to be forever interrupted. Federated America is directing towards deeper levels of "haves" and "have nots" with don't ask don't tell Silence = Death being a military secret only allowed for the "haves" to discuss behind closed doors. The continued harassments being left unnoticed in America says America is uncaring and many countries beyond Federated America already realize America is an arrogant uncaring place to live to never care for individuals judged outside the American military "status quo".

The Bush Administration continual harassments filled with people that concoct schemes of harassment or the deemed "unfortunate enough" to be targeted by American creative military "in action" strategies and viruses for nobody to be meaningful to force individuals into the growing cattle yards of status quo easily manageable to mold people into what someone else wants someone to be controlled by the best evil people of the Bush Administration of who they are. Could you imagine being molded by the Bush Administration strategies to be a part of their destruction of the world? It is literally a nightmare today living in Federated America of business as usual dismal while the underground scheming of the Bush Administration slowly directs people to be intentionally mismanaged to feel hurt and pain of their torturous ways destroying life and unable to tell them to stop. How can anyone do anything let alone the best someone can be under constant duress of the harassments? Be all you can be in a constant state of shock within a military controlled environment becoming more intrusive in our lives today is more silence and more death. Many today are wounded or ill in Federated America today getting worse because of the Bush Administration giving a "meantime" of agendas in constant don't ask don't tell limbo and excruciatingly painful heading in the wrong direction for individuals being wasted in our lifetime seeing ourselves as people suffer.

HIV clinical trials using military style recruitment tactics to either be harassed or be harassed to be recruiters within a community to conveniently recruit more people into a pit of internal war and disease is an enormous weight of decimation pitting one against another. Being militarily owned, operated, or played to be on a ugly level of lost in time is a bad way and no way out is tragic living in America of no choices. Time in long stints of interruption of manmade disease or manmade Federated hate crimes involving don't ask don't tell mantra mentalities to miss the best of an individual can offer trying to live is the worst offensive crime against humanity forever growing worse today furthering us from God not being the "best humans" anyone could be in love and forgiveness. We need to grow and cry for better reasons alive today and not dead to get to heaven above or on planet earth. The Bush Administration growing us stagnant is so sad in America today being manipulated in the land of "opportunities" in a round-a-bout deviant ways diverted or interrupted omitted are opportunities of the Bush Administration and company destroying justice for all our memories to be more than bits and pieces dismembered by right winged freedoms of a right to many lives aborted. Too bad America does not allow better remembrances to give more meaning to life of feeling the Bush Administration's despair tactics to translate into healing instead of growing tired within their military gap uncaring of heartache tugging out of nowhere of lost time of what could be all anyone could be given freedom and equality in a healthy and robust environment void of forced silence.

We could easily imagine growing together to grow past the insane mentality of "tolerance" of the few harboring hate to be accepting and not mere tolerance. The Bush Administration and co-spnsors of promises unfolding to unleash an avalanche of hate to destroy acceptance by unleashing new HIV/AIDS type massive epidemics for many to be forced tolerant of any situation the Bush Administration and company bestows upon us will be a perpetual time of sadness. Forcing acceptance of a distributed disease into the body is a waste of humanity. Why do we have to endure so much pain to feel? We desperately need to end the agendas before it is too late and we wish we would have listened to end the silence. Federated America is a scary place, and if we did not have to live in tolerance of the Reagan and/or the Bush eras of hateful selfishness tearing us apart still today putting individuals into compartments and labeled trying not to be scorned or torn apart then life would be more meaningful in time better spent to be more productive than human products molded to be tolerated today ambiguity of hate crimes apparent. Federated America harassing innocent citizens to be the way they want us to be forcing us against our will to be torn apart never will close the gap of the way nature intended us to be moving our feet together in dance to progress naturally.

The continued business optimization of virus creations and mutations in monopolized time continuing horrific scientific outcomes on selected humans will never amount to much no matter how much time is spent in American harassment mode to feel good about creating internal horrors optimizing furthering along idyllic concepts of perpetuating war. The Bush Administration and company using arsenal products in metal and viruses creating more businesses as usual and status quo forcing more infiltration and confusion into living is excruciatingly inhumane and massively destructive. Metal and viral weapons being stored in confines in warehouses being distributed to enter the human bodies in spirit is dismal to depart capsulized deteriorated of self worth chipped away by fear of health ramifications.

Immunity complications with accompanying discrimination and stigma to carry more burden cannot possibly be a friendly fire of the heart to carry that much weight to be content with Federated America hurting people. Self defense in voice should be equality today and Silence = Death controlling today is far from fair of the internal loss sad in frustration and not much to say controlled to carry on the way we are manipulated to be unopposed and internally silently disenfranchised. America should be given a chance for individuality to control rage into betterment of feeling no pain to heal out in the open, yet unfortunately under Silence = Death strategies of the Bush Administration and co-sponsors of death and dying life is excruciatingly difficult.

The escalating gaps in genetic laboratory viruses strains the heart of HIV in varying degrees and virulent attributes furthering an agenda of forced populations desolate growing in numbers on the street in pain and no way to feel outside of confines of military ceilings. Recently the Department of Defense occupied HIV research, and as a result an escalation of business ventures have sprouted to be a part of the big business of HIV/AIDS. On the other hand, the outlets to describe pain and loss in Federated America today are next to none since organizations such as Act-Up and Gay Mens Health Crisis have virtually closed their doors in silence. The remaining outlets of Federated America are places of infiltration, disease distribution and covert documentation venues of Patriotic idiotic "Acts" documenting feelings to create more destruction and despair to stop life and perpetuate the concept and realities of HIV/AIDS. The strains of HIV in a "pick and choose" new world order of business in varying degrees of hate and control in a vial on the shelf is not much unless someone is one of them "me too" people with "rights" to government and company resources that enjoys seeing people suffer for tailor made pockets of green.

Love and repression are no strangers to awareness of surroundings that denies growth in love. A love connection being denied communication to connect by individual expression lost in time by an amputation of life and limb struggles is not worthy of America that is a pit of despair. America under the Bush Administration is diseased from the top down getting worse all the time from their constant mutating and deforming society to be a battle ground of the Republic with no song or joy to be alive unencumbered and unrestrained to announcing love should not be so difficult. America is ruining so much to be so little repressed feelings. The Bush Administration denying Gay intimate companionship is living without any reason to live except to be at constant battle alone. G. Bush Jr. Is a divider not a decider. What reasons are there to live in denial of the truth? What true joy of intimacy in life to truly fall in love with life unless there is truth? Where is the joy in growing emotionally to be attached to life and love if living is not felt to the bone with chills up the spine in awareness of happiness living in transparency and not fear of living behaved and controlled until death due us part with a cross-species infection in the spine and no backbone to stand up for the truth regarding the HIV/AIDS charade?

Nature allows us to realize spirituality and no matter how much hate and despair is tossed at us our health should be our number one priority to remain spiritually active intact together. Why does love need to battle hate since love is a peaceful realm and being outnumbered by hateful strategies of a different judgmental animal viciously crumbling love into ruins as a game is pure ignorant evil? Why not just hate battle hate instead of hate growing into closet space of love not able to have movement or a Gay voice pronounced dead upon arrival at the starting point? Trapped surrounded by hateful targeting practices is not healthy for anyone anywhere at any age anytime. Living is just so tiring being targeted just for being Gay Out Loud and proud to fight the battle of HIV/AIDS tired of the battle being so deadly lop-sided. An Indian in societal prison left to reservations of love being isolated everywhere reverts to nature to love and wonder if humanity will ever come around to change the song birds tune to love songs out of the environmental caged open out in the wild together in our own back yards.

Breeding so-called New World Monkeys for HIV/AIDS research to murder in cages is the worst of the worst of chromosome for chromosome nonhuman primates and humans can be identically matched using diabolical scientific genetic engineering life to be spent in cages from genetically engineered viruses to a test tube. Besides the fact they have the cure for HIV/AIDS, and besides the fact the Bush Administration and co-sponsors needlessly murder primates and nonhuman primates alike with lab born viruses the need for even one human in a clinical trial is compounding more death and dying exponentialy by pure ignorant evil chromosome for chromosome.

No matter how intense the hate in sterility of hate warm to winter of timely death the seasons need desperate awareness for the leaves to stay. The diseased judicial branches of American government today under the Bush Administration and co-sponsors removing life should be required to leave the American human branches to heal human nature. The parasitic adventures of corruption forcing legislating judicial footnotes to drop bombs onto society to stay will root twisted trees to fall in mass numbers leaving no winter only freezing winds to freely blow more and more untimely deaths the Bush Administration's hate sowing needs to be dug out to get to the root of the problem to untwist the branches and the trees. HIV/AIDS is every war past and present to be built upon to culminate more designer wars and more designer diseases and more designer deaths. A folded American flag put upon a fallen troop to be a hand me down off a plane is AIDS more of the agonizing time of living today as a civilian under scrutinizing stigma and don't ask don't tell wounded and fighting to live in and around slow are "fags" folded over many coffins of friends and family before dying a worse war of a lifetime.

With more troops past and present dying out of plain site of a personal untold story are also civilians of don't ask don't tell HIV/AIDS as cause of death in the obituaries of an untold cold war of AIDS leaving us alone in society before during and after death and dying. The Bush Administration and co-sponsors of AIDS designing cold wars craving more American troops at attention to be sent overseas to be warm murdered cold will cause more hurt and pain to be installed into society and consequently put more fear into society. Allowing more pain and suffering to be transported by plane back to America is cold hearted allowing for more distribution systems of don't ask don't tell frustrations of HIV/AIDS coinciding traumas never to compare war stories. A mainstay in America being manipulated by the Bush Administration and co-sponsors of war of don't ask don't tell Silence = Death allowing for fear factors to be transported into society is society becoming more ugly to be easily twisted and manipulated allowing good energy to fade and be replaced by measly designs in an never ending psyche of cold.

The Bush Administration of control to cold is more sickness, death and dying and when supporting our troops as an enigma scattered could be for starters subtracted joining with PFLG (Parents and Friends of Lesbians and Gays) as an organization of support of all troops Gay or Straight in plight to fight society could gain more physical heartfelt bodies to embrace not as an enigma for the truth to prevail strong instead of political grievances. We need more moral support to subtract coffins out of the fold to end don't ask don't tell immoral mantra of Silence = Death and cold heartedness joining unwillingness to "comply" militarily. Halloween razor candy is HIV/AIDS to transpire horror in how could anyone do such a thing mantra creating fear of how could the government and co-sponsors of disease distribution hide such bitter and spite to be sweet to swallow their poisonous apples of life altering gags to bag dead troops? Poisoning goodies has been a mainstay since the Regan years of HIV/AIDS to Tylenol to Gulf War Syndromes and beyond toxic shocks into the body being altered spiritually by fear of a love canal in a heart pumping blood being brutally beaten sad by government and industry pollution.

A government and co-sponsored packaged deal to decimate the body and soul is a raw cold day at a brutal burial sight to tuck away in scrap mental memories fragmented and torn to remember dead. The smell of HIV/AIDS in the graveyard is bitter sweet loss below and above ground with residue under flesh of loss rotting and fingers scratching the coffin of tears inside out seeping into the ground water. Life to be polluted again and again and again causing more pollution to recycle fragments of life lost onto the ground to remember deep seep into the soul. America is a wasteland of virtually no reality. A nightmare of unforeseen trauma about to happen and no sustenance for the soul always on guard and always targeted and always isolated and always harassed for future targeting for more harassments and more surreal garbage. America is a waste yet people are not America. Humanitarian is far from America land of wasted lives and advertising blood crossed and double crossed by genetics splicing the heart.

My defiance is so strong against needless death and dying my tears have ingrown inside to grow against the American grain of more food and less people of friends and family afar, dead and nearby unable to connect in Silence = Death starving for life to begin instead of always ending. Hateful repression tactics of the Bush Administration and co-sponsors of the HIV/AIDS charade creating a multitude of Broke Back mountain of tears and fears is not worth America, yet is worth people. America like the Patriot Act giving unwanted nourishment by distributing death and dying co-mingled as America is far from any American's dream except the few the not so proud to be American of the Bush Administration and co-sponsors of disease distribution. Disease distribution channels as a copyright day after day deliberating "me too" industry viral products of the same crap to put on the medical shelves is creating an America nobody would ever dream about far from patriotic and far from America being a safe or sane place to live. The Bush Administration and co-sponsors of the HIV/AIDS charade perpetuating ignorant and dangerous awareness messages of virtual threats of do this don't do that don't ask don't tell can't you read the signs illiterate garbage while people suffer and die needlessly by the signs in and of the times is more impoverishing crap to digest.

Where is real love or societal transparency to be real to love of self stymied to be loved? The Bush Administration agendas and repressive strategies to down low someone or low self of esteem someone trying to get uphill everyday repressed by feelings of societal thoughtlessness and complacency is America today on the "down low" low rent and corrupt. The Bush Administration and co-sponsors causing society to be corrupt as a militant society of war and disease gossip to real famine the souls Hitler style victims being removed one by one or a bunch at a time is such a wasteful living agreement. Broke Back mountain of tears and fears with hate crime bloodshed and viruses overhead with war undertow and shit and more proof of the crap onto the shit to be silenced is shitty shitty bang bang we are dying waist high in death and destruction of disease and war.

It is sexy being protected because of love and intimacy sexy to grow stronger in love united in complete communication of the truth. The Bush Administration's concept of protection is a culture of safety for themselves causing so much pain and destruction in the world. There is no true love of nation today under the Bush Administration constantly abusing love of nation by trying to perpetuate an illusion of protection in color coded animation using viruses and bombs to climb their labeled ladder of success towards world control patting themselves on their back slippery slopes. If Americans truly loved country then we would pull together and impeach the Bush Administration before more friends and family are further abused and hurt physically and emotionally. 911 emergency theater costing many lives to stage the Bush Administration as the all elusive "decider" is not honest nor transparent, and in fact, the Bush Administration is an abuser of love playing on American emotions of American history of family pulling together to console each other in a time of crisis not to be further torn apart by a dishonest "decider" and no President with only one oar in the water.

The inequality of growing a world of business executives with mean hateful streaks and greed popping off more viral content to create more ultra wealthy trust funds will create more torturous care and will never allow true healthy understanding of what matters most to flourish in the world not compartmentalize wild is nature and prisons are for humans wild for nature. Time should be more than an anomaly to wonder why time is wasting creating new HIV strains unhealthy all the way around time lost flying HIV off the shelf to say cross-species infections just happen. When will the HIV/AIDS insanity stop vicariously from one hand to a syringe to be less alive vicariously through another wishes death and dying to feel power?

Housing will always be a project. It is shelter from the storm of war and disease created by corruptness of the Bush Administration that is creating more blight by spending down our resources with mere discrimination always intentional by the housing authority to degrade people from two cups and a string unable to communicate from a place of authoritarian blight. A respect storm is the needed fixer upper to clean up the mess of things we call dispersement overseas in troops and money and disease dispersement to the troops on the ground in America and around the world unable to communicate. The "system" does not support HIV/AIDS. Government is perpetuating HIV/AIDS the system the trap of nightmares dosing and doping individuals with crap and orders to obey the system to get services more often than not rendering people worse off less of life and living.

Does anyone realize how many filaments of healing are needed to fill the holes created by destructive political strings pulling every which way but loose the person to be apart of America unwillingly and unknowingly creating war and disease for millions? How filaments are remnants reverted to create more holes in more people at war wounded huddled together in structure being judged without a heart not being deep enough to survive. Shame on America that allows the Bush Administration to be in the business of selling souls to the devil to convince American life is better controlled and not worth saving worldly lives.

Microsoft is intentionally neglecting people because technology is insanely flawed and not remarkable. Remarkable is a voice and unremarkable is not American government and co-sponsors intentionally putting people into traps and cages that has abilities to shut the person up beyond flesh and blood personification denouncing the one way see thru mirror of upside down HIV/AIDS awareness of cages. The environment of nature is omnipresent and not mere mechanical metropolitan serendipity charged gatherings of no real relief or substantial meaning to the massive numbers of people living with HIV/AIDS in cities and towns now more old world gossip centers of disconnect and suburbia. Today is not lending way to appreciate the joy of nature everywhere to remember the day without fallen soldiers here and abroad as memorable. The Great Barrier Reef is mesmerizing though dying faster than the death and dying exuded from the collar stiffs of colorless expression barriers that shift and create more death and dying under water and ground recognized unsalvageable ignored and in plain sight of day repertoire of Silence = Death.

Silence = Death and a rolling stone gathering no moss mantra of the Bush Administration and oil corporations steam rolling along day after day without respect for nature's moss as a source of good green moisturizing steam rising in the morning sun captured by a snap shot of beauty to the eye and heart. Today under the destructive practices of the Bush Administration and co-sponsors of death and dying the moss is being rolled over and over until it is just a fraction of its size unrecognizable to the eye removing mostly for surety purposes removing sensuality and sexuality of touch from our lives. The Bush Administration and co-sponsors are rolling all over us today in a wrong direction of awareness friction removing the green moss we see and feel of beauty and touch real to touch only filaments of memories left behind. The well oiled monster machine of the Bush Administration perpetuating abrasive friction to Global Warming drying our senses void of well healing is sad today how we see the world as a glass system half full or half empty dependent upon the electricity in the political atmosphere magnetizing to hear a pin drop and never sink into the dire reality of the real world.

The rules must change faster than the rolling stone or the Barrier Reef will need an encyclopedic revision expensive in consequences around the world to change the name to rubble unless we collect Silence = Death awareness apparent plain as day to pick up the newspaper to line our garbage cans. What good is forgiveness unless there is awareness of a helping hand along the way to see the Art of a rolling stone with moss as power of caring to heal? It is the helping hand that lulls the ocean and enables the storm not to be so severe of disease and war American style of waste where caring is forgotten today to roll out the cot for others for everyone to sleep safe and sound with dreams of true vibrancy into a deep healing and lulling sleep. Happiness is not true happiness rolling along with the flow today lucky to be alive never safe and sound sad and upside down in the Bush Administration environment of disease and war attack strategies. The totalitarian style Bush Administration abruptness and abrasiveness against a pursuit of happiness requires money to just to avoid their harassments in leverages of powered money mutations of the meaning of habitat for humanity flowing from all directions transforming our environment into an atmosphere of attacks stopping the flow of spiritual healing and peace for all.

Current upstream battles against the current attack strategies of the Bush Administration is wrongful living under toe and thumb where salmon sweep the feet of so-called dignitaries and food is disrespected today in America unwilling to pick ourselves up and start all over again just because we are afraid of the monster that resides in the White House. Americans are unwilling to accept responsibility to live a better life by being more aware of the polluted political environment and impeach the Bush Administration's hate tainting the White House with trapped ghosts. The HIV/AIDS charade is an enormous pit of despair where HIV drugs of mediocrity of good and bad intentionally combined in combination therapy "treatment" to change a person slowly spiritually emotionally and genetically over time is not only intense abuse but misuse of time to destroy the hearts of people labeled HIV/ AIDS as well as friends as family. The Bush Administration deception practices blowing wind thru our heart valves whistling in silence forming no words is a helpless frozen feeling in time not to understand why we are being abused. Abuse stemming from being Gay a minority to AIDS a growing majority with a minority is sad not to be able to live a life in America.

Abuse stemming from the HIV/AIDS charade on many levels and the pharmaceutical HIV/AIDS drugs that follow to the front lines equating Gay as deformed hallucinogenic to be Gay or otherwise from the so-called "norm" is torture to be alive and well in spirit not understanding why hate crimes come from the outside transforming inside bewilderment. Nobody should have to be required to be a citizen of an American infrastructure that currently has installed strategies of attack with long term consequences that are latent and can turn against us on a whim by a hidden twisted political right winged judgement without informed consent to be violently raped of life. Time being wasted struggling to survive and be happy is too much to be constantly sad as an American citizen living around the torture the Bush Administration is deepening their installation environment of war distributing heartache to survivors of their obituary column owned by an installed political infrastructure of real life strategies distributing disease and war.

Disruptions and interruptions allow for grievances to flourish where HIV/AIDS victims awareness is all too aware innately gnawing inside grinds with the sound of sensitivity required to live outside of the political storm of firm hand viruses dictating grievances. The hands on firm hand viruses as a team of war and destruction of the body of the human child far removed from the Bush Administration patting themselves on the back of more evil handy work than anyone can imagine shaking a walking cane at the heavens wondering why me lord. The Bush Administration's infrastructure of no accountability denounces God by delivering bad will and no testament of Silence = Death. Why is it in America the weather is for emotions to be jeopardized, minimalized, or marginalized upon the big microscope of invasion of the Bush Administration body snatchers that believe emotions are not a character trait in a militant society of don't ask don't tell the count of body bags as a gauge of no success in Silence = Death. Why is understanding never put to the test to relax living in the era of the HIV/AIDS a charade ten feet tall to an infant that sees the crops down on the ground under nurtured for the soul. Food is Christ yet the wafer wobbles at the alter of food to mouth unable to voice too weak to imagine the infant lost in Silence = Death not to grow at all too sad and overgrown with deafening silence. Christ did not want to be a spectacle as a looking glass of disbelief and would rather have lived in communion with more people. HIV/AIDS is disbelieve with no societal communion except for a candle light vigil the same disbeliefs of spiritual life on earth.

Christ was torn from the cross in ambition vacant and void to grow food today is the direction of Christ simple always and easily healed today with a voice and action against Silence = Death. Everyone is Christ and if HIV/AIDS is the cross to bare then everyone should be willing to listen to Silence = Death is not a political right to a life to slowly die on the cross to bare. Privacy many times is the mainstay to sexuality and desire to love, yet privacy is not allowed as another strategic alliance to establish abstinence and not a care in the world for HIV/AIDS. Out of sight out of mind literally the soul is being torn apart to be strategically disengaged. Living is everything and money is nothing without a life money is depreciated to the point of disrespect and disaster of time unimportant and down graded to poignancy of time and death of details, and more details tearing down the bodies from the cross manipulated by grievance money. Why hit anyone?

What really constitutes a "high priority"? A stolen dance is jealousy. A stolen body and soul not to dance never should never take place to be happy to dance glorifying abstinence of the elusive right winged party of no healing the ghosts of HIV/AIDS awareness in our closets disrupting and disgusting living around the Bush Administration environment today. Today is being disrupted by more improved upon HIV/AIDS awareness. The evil political party with bats in their belfrys inhabiting houses from their perpetual incubation period of the American White House growing no plants or plans of nature to be seasonally abused. The Bush Administration trying to enhance the disorder of America by disruptive healing with more drama in HIV/AIDS awareness is perpetual murder in motion from a single vaccine or good bad medicine of HIV/AIDS to trumped up awareness is a bad hallucinogenic drug trampling over our senses of love. America is a terrible place to live and die. The face of AIDS puts forth twists in happiness and not to see the effort in smiling thru the pain in America is a million miles away from right winged Christianity. The political ungrateful smile whereabouts everyday protection of nothing becomes more difficult for the innocent self healing from the harsh realities of deceit and meanness of the unholy unhealthy cross of America under the Bush Administration.

Somewhere in the world is an aquarium, amusement park or restaurant being built or planned by water to see fish of all colors of the fish to look from the outside in their natural home divided by a thin real barrier. For what? An experience? If people want an experience try voicing against Silence = Death or being targeted with harassment or targeted with a manmade disease. Everyone sees the disparity, but the people that dress for success in front of the fish sprinkled by big money around the world believing the fish do not see captivity is insane behavior in and of itself the Bush Administration of no captivating character behavior to end HIV/AIDS to enjoy nature more profoundly. Next time at the zoo look into the eyes of seals in captivity and nine out of ten of the seals will have formed a cloud over their eyes. The fabric of life is torn for a reason and many times is self gratification of the amount of money in storage and never enough reason to declare war.

The Bush Administration is in constant photo op mode stature always a million miles away drowning our basic human rights not to be free of the varying degrees of harassment more profound in individual isolation. Even one fish that can spark illumination natural at all levels of nature's pond and happy in a school, but humanly isolated the fish grows fungus even in the most expensive zoo being moved from here to eternity and back handled unmoved in by spirit of the new school of Bush Administration decimating reasoning.

The collection of Art figurines is no different than the imagination to see fish better in nature. Art is a difference in education to imagine a better world without containment facilities. What really is proverbial education in America unable to dissect the true meaning of HIV/AIDS awareness? Do people not understand under funding is not the Art of time lost from AIDS? Art in America is being reversed holy grail of Art lost of Aids dumbfounded against the wall always of time regurgitating the same old crap of death and dying timely day after day of no real imagination to enjoy living Art in nature.

Wait and see the hate will change to transpose our words to more grievance money wasted into dust with more Silence = Death in more days of sweating bullets destroying imagination of living Art to be a dead castaway.

Boring is Bill Gates and George Bush Jr. always gravitating towards themselves whenever their souls say people should be raped of life by their incongruence and haphazard lethal judgmental awareness destroying memories of Hollywood Brad Davis and Rock Hudson legends labeled diseases first on film AIDS death awareness on the streets. America is out of focus and first forward void of respect plastic dead first labeled never a place to grow outside of the dirty layered film of compromises outside of human beautiful body. Could it be Ronald Regan and George Bush Sr. and Jr. with their political biases of a Gay dick in hand as a gun stupid in jack off of no prayers on the prairie today full of Matthew Shepard hate crimes on the fence as "special rights"? Equality is not new, yet regarded in Star Track but to no adventure in America Broke Back Mountain going back in time today as a sign of things to come. We need more healing not more wasted time by grievance money creating inequality futuristic today.

Yee Haw to the mall of no fun adventure better fun in imagination than stand off with guns adventure. Yee Haw love Times Squared in half and Hollywood times of compromises an Idol vote nod off with your head yea or nay a Country Music Television song of all cares and all is good in the country still a vote and still despair in all who cares above and beyond. Church and state hurts many, but HIV/AIDS hurts us all that care for humanity never idolized always a secret and always don't ask don't tell Silence = Death hidden in an idolized song. Trust and love straight or Gay a sanctuary place of dreams. Just because Fred Phelps protestant has hate and animosity to protest towards Matthew Shepard and funerals of the natural Rainbow across the street still does not equate to Fred Phelps right winged judgments never protesting a Catholic Priest of many died of AIDS and so profoundly sad living in America today the closet case.

The Catholic Church is as old as the hills and confused only by the graves on their backs does not mean homosexuality does not have a voice of health free and clear in imagination of love. Gay is not by choice and not perverted or words in groins in agony in conversion programs of nonsense today not to find love. Every time hate is on the right winged license to advertently spread laboratory disease on a plate of irresponsible action is outside and inside paramedics following the aftermath of licences of harm breathing helpless by slurs of sexual deviates not given the best care inside the hospital. Trust is not a value in America today under the corrupt Bush Administration from the norm of homosexuality constantly being removed in body bags and abused as the norm and status quo in America.

Military general 4 star dummies displaying breathless words of death and dying and don't ask don't tell of the violations not recessive HIV/AIDS patients as their right to many lives being destroyed by warlords without a backbone of breath always a dummy in time of abstinent prayers sexless and perverted in premature death denying people love. Gay is not a void. Gay is better than don't ask if you think and don't tell if you do. Time and tea time war should not be worthwhile and don't tell military secrets of the doll downtime will tell time so don't ask a lady secrets of beauty or war just because it ain't mechanical proper spokes between the legs.

America of no respect of the dead living as should be denounced as ghostly confused time never to smell America decaying on the fence denying Matthew Shepard and inhabited AIDS defenseless waiting for more than a cowardly organization called the Bush Administration for emergency help. Healing help of goodness and maternal bedside manners into society is needed. Never wilting is the Gay community strong and respectful to do the best we can under the circumstances the same in equality.

Abused in society but never used in respect beyond mannerisms and behaviors we all denounce the rock and the hard place of sexuality being judged in the bedroom. If only the Bush Administration would leave the Gay community alone to be together without their constant painful harassing bombardments then we would be able to not waste energy to waste to talk back to educate America time and time again of the fallen voluntary Gay radio talk show hosts on the AM dial lost to AIDS in the early morning hours. AIDS is so very costly omnipresent and distraught real distraught misunderstood by time of flesh dead as a flash in the pan. Get it. The whales, elephants and foxes purr and whistle and move as are us in emotional numbers to survive not to be abused a long time ago still today for mevermore by poker hands traveling from east to west and north and south on dirty carpet rides with hazardous bags in storage in flight while holding the pompous bag of the cure of HIV/AIDS. PETA is secluded in nature and Act-Up has virtually been removed. Silence = Death is old hat on top of old politicians balding heads scalping the eagles for nobody to pray Out Loud for survival in their dirty card game of life.

ACT-UP is being deemed a lost cause by the right winged politicians of "winning the war on terror" and ever more PETA is being over run by the same right winged politicians putting more New World Monkeys into cages to allude to HIV/AIDS research dead a flash in the pan resort of advertising death and dying. We are not the last of us not extinct to be mad of Act-Up dwindling as the last to run over road death and dying all too familiar not dead as visionaries of the human race yesterday today and a future of hope for ending HIV/AIDS. Not so stupid to get in a car with a Gay of only dilemmas of environmental harassments trying to untangle confusion and love driving the story home alone to end Silence = Death with friends as family. Alone inside the limit of societal walls when outside the curtains of death and dying are to get home with friends as family. Only life matters outside of the stupid Bush Administration denying life.

Love of self should matter with love of others to drive daisies up real in a habitat for humanity not pushing daisies up by death caused by laboratory disease labeled in plastic coated HIV/AIDS of real suffering. Why have community school unless there is interaction to end Silence = Death of curtains draping over the grave? Iraq and not so disclosed the number yet to die as Americans by the all mighty Bush Administration unwittingly knows all not to well the ill by firm hand calculations of death of human numbers to money to recruit to send to demolish and to bring back home to ma and pa in a bag or on an AIDS Quilt of colors denounced by Bush Administration excuses to "stay the course" of death and dying.

Buried and ruining ma and pa by the born again shop of globalization outnumbering imagination and still no education to end HIV/AIDS and Silence = Death equals no intelligence level registering within the Bush Administration outwardly able to voice Silence = Death is good for morale to don't ask don't tell. HIV/AIDS and Matthew Shepard over the fence defenseless figured hate is a crime without convicting the crime as hate is where we are today of no compassion only hate and crimes. Go figure nothing changes and HIV/AIDS are delusions of still on Broadway someway somehow the messages are not a play of amusement of disease labeled HIV/AIDS today in reversed awareness and no education of pain of the HIV/AIDS charade. Only if yesterday without HIV/AIDS were today and not a playwright in time and not Silence = Death for a new day of education is personal and not climbing young or old towards the light of AIDS candle light vigils. Is there no remembrance of the dead in war of reality of HIV/AIDS wasting valuable time as a purple heart bruised by loss. The war veterans wounded could help the Gay community out of the HIV/AIDS charade as assisted living for true hospice care and habitat for humanity healing on site to live as true Americans at such an early age today of all Americans subjected to clinical veterinary aviary caged barbaric care today in Military America.

Top or bottom has no privacy today to be real with a hard man good to find. If only there were no gaps in communication then explosive love would be private without war of Patriot Acts intruding on our lives to be judged on the edge of infringement disregarding totally the con Patriot Acts. Con Patriot Acts intruding on our oasis of frenzy is far removed from taboo scared fear run and hide and seek and be destroyed are pet names of the Bush Administration without the love of animals. Free at last in a prayer dream for a better tomorrow for hope on a wing and a prayer. Free at last for the least of us still trying at least to be alive to have decency in and out of the cage of no respect in America of no lease in life controlled.

Education is more attractive than the illusions of religion of no substance only more priests with HIV/AIDS and more politically polished in grace throwing stones in glass houses to quiet the Silence that equals Death and starvation of spirituality. Hate is not a family value. The HIV/AIDS charade ruined a zest for sincerity for humanity being replaced by bitterness and painful medicine intake with food. God does not damn it the food God damn it is the interruptions that have stolen our identities and lives to the HIV/AIDS charade of bogus treatments and government and pharmaceutical companies demanding to take your own medicine. Long stints of life interruptions with fear as a mainstay diet to Silence = Death is not living or dreaming of equality when we have done nothing wrong having same sex equal relationships.

Healing comes from transparency of the rain not the forest thru the trees of government and co-sponsors of elusive HIV/AIDS advertised with cures yet to be found in a needle and a haystack in the rain forest of nature. The HIV/AIDS charade of self destruction making love is the worst lie ever since we could heal ourselves in nature to be better than discrimination of love. If only the Bush Administration and co-sponsors of the big business of HIV/AIDS would stop the releases of laboratory diseases called HIV/AIDS and release the laboratory obtained cures for the various mutations of disease called HIV/AIDS then we could easily see the rain and the forest for what it means to heal nature and humanity.

Destroying the rain forest is Global Warming of overload of polluting nature with laboratory made viruses created by erratic behaviors of government and co-sponsors of HIV/AIDS to be evolution of humans and disrespect to pollute nature. Evolution takes millions and billions of years. Hopefully the Bush Administration will not be a complete 8 years. God is healing and why allow church and state to interrupt our lives with pain and suffering as a combined entity of church and state spitting on God out of body or accountability of reversed prayers actively interrupting our lives with pain and suffering always stemming from the HIV/AIDS charade mutating togetherness deformed. The HIV/AIDS charade is complete abandonment of identity and life beyond the Bush Administration and co-sponsor's growing strategies of daily interruptions causing more pain and suffering.

When will the hands of interruptions stop so healing can turn back their miserable hands in our time for good riddance today of more than a fair trade to get our complete lives back for inclusiveness as more than betterment on the road to healing? Compromises are not security under the Bush Administration business hands concocting pain, mistrust, corruption and fear with and without God to respect the hurricane of the Bush Administration dismantling God today not found in church and state running over our lives. The Bush Administration of war and violence as their platform is so sad living during their time of hate times seventy compounded by church and state interrupting our lives.

Designing cloned animals and designs of cloning people judged of worth as a novelty item is the wrong direction to bless food for spirituality of body and soul. The misuse of Genetics not to produce more plants and vegetables and grains is an agenda the Bush Administration and co-sponsors of death and dying neglect moreover everyday for more control over the world to become a sad lost world. Genetically engineering cells of animals and humans incorporating viruses to gene alter "populations" over time creating more discriminating tastes while researching rapidly cloning animals by the same genetic engineering enthusiasm is not to sustain life but rather the Bush Administration and co-sponsor's agendas to discriminate life and mold "fitter families" as the status quo of eugenic agendas.

The Bush Administration and co-sponsors living in their dangerous plastic superiority complex bubbles in pollution. The misuse of genetics is creating more differences than anyone could imagine the future instead of healing today to be all we can imagine gracefully. Why are we suppose to shut up shut in and isolate away as a gateway to internalize a prayer needing a wing and a prayer to compute out loud? Why not living prayers to live creating a normal environment instead of an AIDS quilt so disheartening in normalcy?

It is time we put some real Americans in the White House instead of counter culture right winged hypocrites that are destroying our foundation and calling themselves model citizens with a right to our lives when all they have ever done was manipulate, destroy and control their way to be a "strong arm" in selfishness murdering humanity decimating to a fault anyone that cares about a right to life. Where are the real leaders that realize the importance of humanity to grow in peace accords, and why and how it gotten this bad where American leaders destroy citizens to be "subjects," "cohorts" or "subpopulations" endemically modeled and labeled in disease and labeled graves on sight?

Science projects confusing birth with political rights and American leaders paving the way to be their way or the highway today in the White House of harms way growing stronger is not even fit to be a nation of human beings of unequal birth rights. The CDC HIV/AIDS estimates pertain to the United States and the administration along with the other HIV/AIDS charade players have separate agendas in different parts of the world as well as with different targeted populations to be hit hard dependant upon the political agenda.

The different "populations" targeted and labeled dependent on the political agenda is the same everywhere comprised of ill-willed selfish objectives far from democracy and further away from humanity and peace. Why not target the moral majority if targeting with disease is the only option to control populations with set behaviors tagged with various intentional infections and entrapment of HIV testing, stigmatization, and intervention to clear a path for more shared fair playing ground of real estate wars with more true expressive behaviors of reversed equality and less Silence = Death? And maybe start with the Fred Phelps congregation "subgroup" that invades AIDS victim's funerals carrying signs of immoral judgment that defaces the congregation and spits on the graves of innocent victims lost in excruciating pain? All it would take would be a few stigmatizing HIV infections mysteriously emerging within their congregation, similar to the mysterious infections that emerged in the Gay community during the Reagan years, and the agony would rattle their lives the same equally, yet unfortunately create another "population" considered "high risk" to be lessened and never informed of the true spiritual power of people being denounce by church and state.

The Bush Administration and the immoral majority are inflicting death by empowering and controlling science to be manipulative, yet standing on ceremony and publicity stunts designed at holier than thou attributes intended to offset any notions they would be part of such painful infliction they religiously depict to be sent from God as retribution. Not only is the Bush Administration and the religious right hate mongers, liars and anti-American, but worse in serving up God human mutations guised by some as evolution from laboratory scientists diseasing bodies. In reality the Bush Administration and the hate mongers are devil worshipers in disguises spreading diseases of mistaken identities in the name of one word HIV/AIDS.

The horrendous atrocities being silently draped over humanity where remorse is left in the dust and replaced with strategic business plans and agendas of hidden torture yet to be revealed to be cleansed on earth by God and healed from diseases being sent from laboratories not of God. What is moral and spiritual about extinguishing human life? Extinguishing human life is a criminal activity opposite of peace in God and caring of fellow human beings, and is a breeding ground for corruption to grow in hate that spreads similar to a bad infection always void of affection unless it is brought home to share the suffering to be part of family enlarging sadness misunderstood in silence. Why hate Gays to death? Why hate anyone to death when God has our best interests at heart to realize truth to give meaning for life to grow unencumbered and grow healing of human family? What is missing to be revealed to be cleansed on earth is the truth. The obstacles of political agendas invading our lives on the most remote physical and spiritual levels needs exposure to breathe true health care to truly understand the power of all types of healing.

The maniacal and intentional disease causing government and partners in crime destroying life as we know it with disease, HIV testing traps, stigma ramifications, targeting spirituality, is something that needs the entire planet earth to behave responsibly and embrace together as spiritual beings if not for the purpose of saving all of our lives against the government and company owning firm hand viruses controlling our lives in fear moving away from trust.

Sloth oaths of the Bush Administration maggots is the ticket today of no real meaning to the Bush Administration harassing entire communities and abusing the communications system to corrupt society. Oath could be the truth to convey a sloth is an animal and a maggot is an insect, but today violent immune complications from the HIV/AIDS charade is creating problems and funeral processions agitating life with no recourse to heal the violence of Silence = Death. The Bush Administration's deceptive practices as tickets to life could be shredded if America was allowed a good vision with communication needing transparency to be seen. The law of the land has changed under the Bush Administration promoting deception creating violence. Medical school or Law school are opposing forces yet the same time spent learning a trade secrets of malpractice deception one way or the other wasting time opposing views of the deceptive ticket to life the Bush Administration is trying force into our communication processes.

Medical laboratories genetically engineering viruses to harm entire communities being targeted with communications strategies to convey people are bad to validate illnesses needs more lawyers in America today than ever with a heart and less scientists and medical research practicing with half a brain to intentionally hurt people with abusive physical violence that Lawyers do not practice. Accountability is all but extinct in America with a deceptive ticket to life to not ask doctors and scientists questions under oath within an infrastructure of the Bush administration punishing people that want the truth to stand under scrutiny saving time and lives. Don't ask don't tell Silence = Death and paper to legislative viral machine guns out of nowhere shredding people to shred their lives to tinker toy soldiers camouflaged in betrayal of Christmas lights up the Bush Administration's eyes of deception infiltrating people to be dissected and manipulated highlighted on the news without style or grace isolated from friends.

Juxtaposed and disposition could be the same in the same space in time if human disposition were not so selfish in nature. The violation in ownership of meaning is rot in the current White House hall of frame. We have a say in our lives, but we are forced not to be taken seriously of anything because of the current American disposition of war at all costs. The disposition of the evil Bush Administration uttering juxtaposed is contraire to love of all people in the room. Gays cannot just exist in peace because of a government hateful disposition and fear of love. People need love and not politics and that is the problem of the Bush Administration's misuse of genetics.

Global warming, New World Monkeys, Knock Off Mice, Heterogeneity, Genetically engineered NIH mini-pigs, Genetically engineered viruses, Cloned and Re-cloned viruses and live viruses sent through the laboratory technique of recombination to cross-species transplant into humans and animals and removed and cloned to be re-transplanted again and again into humans and animals with biocontainment buildings standing by in the name of the Bush Administration's own terror is the hidden reality and just a partial listing of the Bush Administration's hidden agendas. The Bush Administration has gone wild in delusional hype of a superiority and discrimination mess of yesteryear within a fractured time capsule being undressed and re-calculated in behind the door secrets, and in science labs to be yet another monster to be slowly unfurled or rapidly infused into the environmental ecosystem and humanity and never brought up to speed into the now or no future living around the Bush Administration's White House of horrors of deception, bigotry and beyond.

HIV testing and Barrack Obama does not compute to get a point across. Barrack Obama is an advocate for HIV testing yet Barrack Obama has family ties in Africa and HIV testing is a death trap without the cure made available there is no pleasing political incongruities. Come on please at what point do we cross the line to spirituality and not face the same blinding colorless motions of no change in reality? Shame on the people that bargain to the point of no return in the HIV/AIDS charade. The Bush Administration is hell on earth and selling political compromises to the Bush Administration is colorless supporting HIV testing that has no point other than a lifetime of control. When can anyone be separated today from the decimating crap of the right winged political America brimming with secrets and lies that affect all of our lives? A foundation of separate food for oil giving no whey on a platter in our face starving for relief in separation from the repressive Bush Administration withholding the truth.

Money should be played not a gamble but to experiment spiritually in a good way with life to find peace. What or where is the point to equality a mere stripe around the world equating to Global Warming? Gross is America good are people wanting to be together more than a stripe on our backs under the Bush Hitler years cold as hell. The game of colors and words in Bush Administration America means we are controlled. America is all about compromises so life has no real meaning. Communication misses the point to the meaning of life in compromises that bog us down in crap of the Bush Administration with no respect for life. Reaching out is one thing but nature's colors on words to convey compromises and plastic allegiances because of compromises is another living without nature of color. Viewing nature gives more meaning to color and words with no compromises to conceal the meaning of life. If the Bush Administration had their druthers to get their hate across they certainly wood spray paint trees green to deceive people another day. Inspiration is turning coffee into hops and grains for available food for everyone is fed up on the ground of deceit and no food. A wing and a prayer since life is a crap shoot to get around the meaningless barricades put up with the Bush Administration of what options do any of us have in their game of distance from the soul for food?

The best compromise bitter sweet humor today sad is blue fabric on a person from the waist up getting out of a car and yawning at the same time heading into a Gay bar. See cars and oil are boring. There are no excuses for life not to grow and no excuses to allow extinction just because the Bush Administration barricades growing into gaps growing into blockaded communication. Back burner issues should be eliminated. The Bush Administration's fear of mind expansion frustrates and terrorizes the monarchy of taxes and barricades of a seamstress of songs of the times of stress and strife hopefully realizing the plight of a seamstress of hope.

Transportation may be ahead of its time in cars and oil destroying the environment as a cruel means of transportation of few choices, but behind the times in repairing unnecessary traps of repairs and no healing stuck in a car caught in traffic. Ease of transportation could be enjoyable without so many cars barricading life by dreaming about money to get into a car a detour from life abysmal getting from A-Z and no real awareness of hope in between to ease the pain caught in the Bush Administration system of no mind expansion of levitating transportation lessening accidents and violence. HIV/AIDS is upside down awareness today giving certain big business contributors hope to continue the HIV/AIDS charade with oil, automobile, and pharmaceutical industries hope for tomorrow furthering barricading life from reality and pure ignorance in what awareness and education should encompass towards togetherness.

HIV/AIDS encompassing upside down mental health issues educating in fear and terror awareness for tomorrow's disasters not only excludes hope but replaces hope with stress and road rage. The dictionary needs revised to correct right is wrong for America under the right winged Bush Administration constantly making wrong handed turns directing business to flow and chart territories being built by channeling under ground money above the fray into corruption of awfully big business of HIV/AIDS a lie.

The underworld of the Bush Administration distributing their dirty computerized chemical money into their corrupt system of up and down and all around good guy Bush deception reversed macro economics into our lives as the status quo is not fun watching the 4th of any month, or year or second fade into quarantined body time folded in half by genetically engineered viruses to be one eighth of a life stigmatized, traumatized and sent into an early grave. How come there is not more of an outcry to end dismal to get on with our lives in health? Being Gay from a family of liberals and conservatives where my blood brother is conservative and unfortunately under the Bush Administration's demise of humanity is a train wreck never to collide with the truth of being a Christian brother to realize people are not disease. Too bad the Bush Administration is so corrupt that nobody can survive in good will and testimony to destroy Silence = Death giving way to communicate and heal.

Can anyone imagine the number of individual horror stories that never reach the surface in America perpetuating HIV/AIDS labeled the "special people" arguably without "special rights" or any rights whatsoever infected and left gasping for air? What about equality? What about the genetically engineered viruses that were given to the Gay man in Boston and after months and months of agonizing pain the Gay man gave up clinically and was dismissed from the "system" to die alone spiritually bankrupt is America. Another situation where a woman (not detailed in this manuscript) was given several genetically engineered viruses then her face rotted away or the genetically engineered virus construct with cereal grains. Nobody wants to hear about those ordeals in America today being quarantined from reality. Names and labels and constructs around a constitution with no bill of rights withstanding is sadly being mistaken in America today of mislabeled identity. The hills are alive as mortals trying to illustrate Art to live as people not to be sold as special rights caught in between cement around a rock and a hard place to live in a crevice alive abused by the Bush Administration and their strategies perpetuating harassing diseases and war silencing humanity.

The HIV/AIDS charade never emerges into the light of day means the Bush Administration does not need to confront the American Constitution or the Bill of Rights is wrong unused covered in molding rights of no freedom of speech and no real American remembrances of innocent people being buried in cement. Buried in cement for being a Gay person labeled HIV/AIDS is the Bush Administration abusing and torturing their dirty little "special rights" they hideaway in their dirty gigantic laundry closets of games they play being mentally ill putting needles into dolls.

It is so sad so many people die because the Bush Administration cannot be made responsible for their hate crime actions against humanity and we   suffer as citizens abused with no rights whatsoever never to be heard over their consistent pollution gaining perpetual motion of their cowardly injustice terrorist activities never for America to see the light of day. Something real means nothing in America being cemented and shoe boxed in a closet today.

Consistent Bush Administration nature as busy bees being colorless fabric on flesh compromised of no real communication is sad not to communicate Art to voice and put a heart to a face to see humanity good yet being abused today. Not in a closet for an instance any day yet there are physically weak people whom should be allowed to heal more than survive laboratory disease that quarantines in no room space in America fragmented squeezing out good people for no good reason into early graves. The so-called military "Army strong" to scare the pants off Gay behaviors scares many more away one funeral at a time to survive the best anyone can on many levels running and dodging from the American military viral shots. What is the formula to end discrimination for a formula to a mind needing nourishment to digest curiosity being rattled by an over towering mogul spinning overhead behind the times of a baby beginning to dream without product or moguls. Product introduction at such an early age dreaming is sublime mind control to not concentrate on the human dreams at such an early age new. Suffocating dreams of senses causes discrimination of no natural allowances to enter the heart and soul of aromas to dream of not smelling mentholatum behind the times. Natural scents to dream secured and bathed in natural scents lessens the probability of sudden infant deaths to product poison over towering the human enclosed in military environments creating products of control.